Diagnostic Procedures in Nursing Practice

Diagnostic Procedures in Nursing Practice

Jane Vincent Corbett, R.N., M.S.

Associate Professor
School of Nursing
University of San Francisco
San Francisco, California

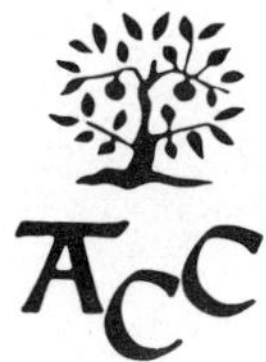

APPLETON-CENTURY-CROFTS/Norwalk, Connecticut

0-8385-1597-5

Notice: Our knowledge in the clinical sciences is constantly changing. As new information becomes available, changes in treatment and in the use of drugs become necessary. The author(s) and the publisher of this volume have, as far as it is possible to do so, taken care to make certain that the doses of drugs and schedules of treatment are correct and compatible with the standards generally accepted at the time of publication. The reader is advised to consult carefully the instruction and information material included in the package insert of each drug or therapeutic agent before administration. This advice is especially important when using new or infrequently used drugs.

83 84 85 86 87 / 10 9 8 7 6 5 4 3 2

Prentice-Hall International, Inc., London
Prentice-Hall of Australia, Pty. Ltd., Sydney
Prentice-Hall Canada Inc.
Prentice-Hall of India Private Limited, New Delhi
Prentice-Hall of Japan, Inc., Tokyo
Prentice-Hall of Southeast Asia (Pte.) Ltd., Singapore
Whitehall Books Ltd., Wellington, New Zealand
Editora Prentice-Hall do Brasil Ltda., Rio de Janeiro

Library of Congress Cataloging in Publication Data

Corbett, Jane Vincent.
Diagnostic Procedures in Nursing Practice

Bibliography: p.
Includes index.
1. Diagnosis. 2. Nursing. I. Title. [DNLM:
1. Diagnosis, Laboratory—Nursing texts. 2. Diagnostic tests, Routine—Nursing texts. QY 4 C789d]
RT 48.C66 1983 616.07′5′024613 82-22723
ISBN 0-8385-1597-5

Design: Jean M. Sabato

PRINTED IN THE UNITED STATES OF AMERICA

To Mary Elizabeth Vincent,
my mother and first teacher

Contents

Preface

As health care becomes more and more technical, the multitude of diagnostic procedures continues to grow. Nurses can become dazzled by the technical details and discouraged about keeping pace with these advances. Yet the nurse's role in relationship to diagnostic testing should continue to focus on the human element. Professional nurses are involved in health teaching, patient preparation, and assessment for adverse reactions to diagnostic procedures. Thus, from a nursing point of view, detailed technical information on diagnostic procedures, using a disease or systems model, may not be the most helpful. Witness the difference in nursing care needed for a patient having a liver biopsy compared to a patient having a liver scan. Although both tests are used to diagnose potential disease in the same organ, there is no similarity in the nursing care.

This book groups particular types of diagnostic procedures so nursing implications can be generalized. For example, nursing care before and after invasive tests is somewhat similar, and much in contrast, to noninvasive tests. Similarly, tests such as sonograms or CT scans have common nursing implications, and endoscopic procedures have common pre- and posttest considerations.

Each chapter of this book can be read independently. Objectives and test questions help the reader focus on some of the most important points. The introductory section gives useful background information (such as radiation hazards common to all x-ray tests) and is followed by a description of each test, purposes, patient preparation (physical and *psychological*), and posttest nursing implications. The rationales for all nursing assessments and interventions are explained. The independent role of the nurse is stressed in setting patient goals and evaluating outcomes.

This book on diagnostic procedures is a companion book to an earlier work, *Laboratory Tests in Nursing Practice*. I hope the reader finds this second book also useful in the practice of professional nursing.

Acknowledgments

Writing a book on such a broad subject as diagnostic procedures requires using information from many sources. Considerable credit must be given to the many references from current nursing literature. I am indebted to the many nurses who have written excellent articles about their experiences.

Elaine Vaughn, Head of Nuclear Medicine and Ultrasound Departments at Kaiser Permanente Medical Center, San Francisco, spent a great deal of time helping me discover what nurses need to know about radionuclides and ultrasound. Other people in the Kaiser Medical Center were also very helpful in freely allowing me to observe various diagnostic procedures and ask a lot of questions. Sunny Holland, R.N., Cardiac Catheterization Laboratory, also at Kaiser, reviewed parts of the manuscript and gave me helpful hints.

My colleagues and students at the University of San Francisco for the past thirteen years have been most helpful as I tried out ideas on them. Mae Paulfrey, R.N., M.S., has been a steadfast and very supportive colleague. Dr. Joan Green, Acting Dean of the University of San Francisco, offered encouragement and support. Students and colleagues from years ago, when I taught at Miami–Dade Community College and Jackson Memorial School of Nursing in Miami, Florida, also contributed to my present knowledge. Many of my personal friends, who are nurses, have also helped in unique ways: Carol Bailey, R.N., M.S. and Terry Corwin, R.N., M.S. deserve special thanks.

My husband, Rod, and our daughter, Rhonda Jane, have been very involved in the many aspects of making this second book a reality. I am most indebted to them for their unending patience and moral support. Debbie Fox, the typist of an earlier book, has also cheerfully worked on this second manuscript. And Jane Licht, at Appleton-Century-Crofts, has been all an author could wish for in an editor.

Diagnostic Procedures in Nursing Practice

CHAPTER ONE

Diagnostic Radiologic Tests

Objectives

1. Describe the difference between fluoroscopy and routine x-ray films.
2. Explain how the four densities of air, fat, water, and bone are represented on x-ray film.
3. Identify three methods to reduce the hazards of radiation from exposure to x-rays.
4. List several important points to teach consumers how to protect themselves from unnecessary x-ray exposure.
5. Identify nursing implications for patients going to x-ray for radiologic study.
6. Identify nursing implications when patients return from radiologic study.
7. Identify radiologic tests that require dye or a contrast medium, and explain how the dye adds additional nursing implications.
8. Name specific nursing actions appropriate in assisting the x-ray technician to get a better portable chest x-ray of a patient in bed.
9. Compare the diagnostic tests covered in this chapter, and identify those tests that cause pain, which often require the use of analgesics.

The first part of this chapter briefly describes the three ways in which x-rays are used in diagnostic testing and how the hazards of radiation can be reduced when diagnostic x-rays are needed. The second part discusses the general nursing implications for preparing a patient for x-ray studies and taking care of the patient after the x-rays are completed. The last part of this chapter gives a description of each of the common x-ray studies and the key nursing implications in caring for the patient before and after each specific test. Although the specific preparation for each test is outlined in this book, the reader is advised to consult with the radiology department regarding the exact protocol to be followed at that particular institution, especially the guidelines given for pre- and posttest care. Most radiology departments have printed guidelines on the preparations needed for each test. The nurse should never hesitate to consult with members of the radiology department if a question arises about what is or is not necessary before a test. In addition, the nurse may need to consult the radiology department when several different tests are ordered for a patient. For example, a radioactive iodine uptake (RAI) test must be done before x-rays with iodine contrast medium. Also, barium studies may make it impossible to do other abdominal tests for a day or two.

Although rare, some radiology departments have a nurse as part of the staff. If a nurse is employed by the radiology department, she or he may have several roles, including: 1) extended temporary floor nurse and guardian, 2) teacher, 3) consultant on how to deal with intravenous bottles, chest tubes, etc., 4) liaison with the clinic staff, 5) team helper for ICU nurse who accompanies the patient to x-ray (Ordronneu, 1980; Maphet, 1981).

In specialized areas, such as an intensive care unit or a small emergency room, nurses may be the first professional to see a person's chest film. Obviously the interpretation of x-rays requires a skilled clinician.[1] The purpose of this chapter is to prepare nurses for the care of patients undergoing x-rays; therefore, there is little emphasis on the interpretation or clinical significance of the findings of x-rays. However, some general information about the clinical significance of a particular type of x-ray is given with each test.

HOW X-RAYS ARE USED IN DIAGNOSTIC TESTS

X-rays were discovered in 1895 by the German physicist Roentgen, who received the first Nobel Prize in Physics (1901) for his discovery. By 1896, the first x-ray machines were in use. Since that time, much has been learned about both the benefits and risks of x-rays or roentgenologic studies. X-rays are electromagnetic radiation of very short wavelengths, which are commonly generated by passing a current of high voltage (from 10,000 volts up) through a Coolidge tube (Miller, 1978). X-rays can penetrate most substances, including human tissues, by strongly ionizing the tissue through which they pass. They cause certain substances to fluoresce and affect photographic plates, qualities extremely useful for diagnostic tests. They are, however, harmful to living tissue. X-rays can alter cells so they cannot reproduce. Consequently, radiation therapy is used to treat various types of cancer. (See Chapter 3 for further examples of the diagnostic and therapeutic use of radiation in the form of radioisotopes.)

At the present time, there are three major ways x-rays are used as diagnostic tests: 1) x-ray films or roentgenograms, 2) fluoroscopy, and 3) tomography. Tests using the first two methods are discussed in this chapter, tomography in Chapter 2.

Roentgenograms or X-Ray Films

Roentgenograms, or x-ray pictures of body structures, are like the negative of a photograph. X-rays that go through the body and the x-rays that reach the film positioned on the other side of the body turn the film black. X-rays penetrate air easily; therefore, areas

[1]See Tinker (1976) and Wilson (1977) written to help nurses recognize some of the major abnormalities revealed by chest films.

filled with air or gas appear very dark on the film. For example, lungs, which contain a lot of air, appear very dark on a plain x-ray film. In contrast, bones or the dyes used as contrast media appear almost white on the film because the x-rays cannot penetrate these substances to reach the sensitive x-ray film. Organs and tissues appear as various shades of gray because they have more mass than air but not as much as bone. For example, heart tissues contain a lot of water and the heart appears lighter on film than say fatty tissues. From the blackest to the whitest the four densities of x-ray are:

1. Air—blackish,
2. Fat—dark gray,
3. Water—lighter gray,
4. Bone—whitish.

Fluoroscopy

In this method of using x-rays for diagnostic purpose, the patient is put in front of an x-ray tube and a fluoroscopic screen is held over the body part to be examined. Recall that x-rays have the ability to make certain substances, such as those used to coat the screen, fluoresce or give off light. As with the roentgenograms, different structures of the body allow different amounts of x-ray beams to project on the fluoroscopic screen. The image remains on the monitor for continuous observation; therefore, any movements in the body can be monitored. For example, as a patient swallows barium, the flow of barium can be monitored on a fluoroscopic screen. Fluoroscopy is also very valuable in cardiac catheterizations to help the physician see the exact position of the catheter in the heart. (See Chapter 7 on cardiac catheterization.) Fluoroscopy is done in the dark so that images of the various densities are seen in sharper outlines. Before fluoroscopy is done the physician puts on goggles with red lenses, which help the eyes adjust to the dark. Fluoroscopy prolongs the time of exposure to radiation, so it is only used when it is deemed very important to observe the change in position of some movement in the body. Videotapes of the fluoroscopic procedure (cineradiography) enable the movements to be studied at later times. Cineradiography is also valuable as a teaching tool.

Tomograms and Computerized Axial Tomography Scans

A tomogram, also called laminagram or planogram, is a special type of x-ray film that is taken with both the x-ray tube and film kept in motion during exposure. The x-ray takes pictures of several different planes of tissues. With each change in the position of the camera, a slightly different level of tissue is in focus. Computerized axial tomography (CT) uses computers, scanners, and tomography to obtain a three-dimensional, cross-sectional view of any body structure. The CT scan is the newest method of using x-rays for diagnostic purpose. (Tomography and CT scans are discussed in Chapter 2.)

REDUCING THE HAZARDS OF RADIATION EXPOSURE

Probably the most important point for the nurse to remember about radiation is that exposure to any type of radiation is cumulative. The nurse must be aware of the serious risks to patients or personnel who are repeatedly exposed to radiation. Some of the risks associated with cumulative doses of radiation are 1) increased chances of developing cancer or genetic damage, 2) sterility, 3) alterations in the make-up of individual cells, and 4) depression of the production of bone marrow. In addition, leukemia is more common in people who use radioactive substances in their occupations. Certainly the amount of radiation in one x-ray is not enough to cause these major problems, but radiation exposure must always be as limited as possible.

The effect on man of any kind of radiation, natural or man-made, is measured in a unit of quantity called rems (*r*oentgen *e*quivalent for *m*an). A millirem is 1/1000 of a rem. Most references estimate that the average American receives 100 to 200 millirems of radiation a year from the sun, cosmic rays, television sets, and diagnostic x-rays. Medical irradiation is probably between 50 to 70 millirems per person per year. The exact amount of radiation, allowed for the general public, cannot be expressed as so many millirems. The general guide of the National Council on Radiation Protection and Measurements (1977) is that all radiation exposure should be held to the lowest practicable level. The permissible levels of radiation incurred under occupational circumstances is 5 rems or 5000 millirems per year (National Council on Radiation Protection and Measurements, 1977). The allowable amount for workers in nuclear plants or in radiology or nuclear medicine departments, however, is not just a simple numerical rule. The formulas used to calculate the allowable radiation exposure for these workers takes into account the lifetime exposure of workers. People who work with radiation must wear badges to monitor the exact amount of exposure to ensure that these limits are not exceeded. Nurses do not need to wear badges because they are not routinely exposed to radiation sources. However, because radiation is cumulative through life, it is reasonable for the nurse to limit exposure to as little as possible, in all situations where radiation is being used. For example, see the discussion in Chapter 3 on handling urine when radionuclides are used for diagnostic tests. The nurse should also help make sure that patients have maximum protection.

Some readers may remember the fluoroscopy machines used in shoe stores before the 1950s. A parent could see, with delight, that the child's shoe was a perfect fit. Yet the risk of this procedure far outweighed the benefit.

At one time, dental x-rays were frequently used for screening purposes. Consumers are now being advised that one should refuse to allow routine dental x-rays every six months, especially for children (Mongeau, 1979). When dental x-rays are needed, one should ask if the machine has a focusing adaptor, which restricts the beam size. Also, the public needs to be taught that lead aprons should be worn even for dental x-rays.

Communitywide use of chest x-rays has been used to screen for tuberculosis and cancer. Routine chest x-rays for tuberculosis are not commonly done anymore, unless there is a reason to suspect the disease.

Based on the risks, benefits, and costs of x-rays as screening devices for cancer, the American Cancer Society's (February 1980) latest recommendation for chest x-rays is to drop the x-ray as a screening device for cancer. The annual chest x-rays, which used to be recommended for early detection of lung cancer, are not deemed worthwhile—even with early detection, lung cancer is still very resistant to cure. Reducing questionable chest x-rays helps eliminate unnecessary radiation exposure. (The American Cancer Society (ACS) feels that more attention to the prevention of smoking is a better way to attack the problem of lung cancer.) The newest guidelines for breast x-rays are covered in the ACS 1980 report on mammograms. Mammograms were widely used in the early 1970s, but again, the use of x-ray as a screening device has been reevaluated in terms of benefits versus risks. (See the discussion on mammograms later in this chapter.)

Wilson (1977) has suggested three questions that need to be asked before a patient is exposed to x-rays:

1. Is the x-ray clearly necessary for the patient's well-being?
2. Are there previous x-rays available or other tests that would serve the same purpose?
3. If x-rays are necessary, is everything being done to assure the lowest possible radiation dose?

Time, distance, and shielding are three ways to offer radiation protection. For example, the time of exposure to x-rays should always be as short as possible. Fluoroscopy is not done if a simple x-ray film will suffice—exposure is shorter with a traditional x-ray. Keeping a distance from the x-ray machine is a second way to avoid radiation exposure. Thus, all personnel should leave the x-ray room when x-ray studies are being done. Occasionally, a nurse may be asked to help with some x-ray procedure being done at the patient's bedside. If the nurse must be involved in the procedure, then shielding is important. Shielding, (the third method of protection from radiation) involves the use of lead as a barrier to the x-rays, e.g., lead aprons and sometimes lead gloves. The walls of the x-ray room are also shielded with lead, as are containers for radioactive materials.

It is sometimes difficult for health personnel to remember that x-rays are present because they cannot be seen, heard, or felt. There is a type of monitor that gives an audible beep when the wearer is exposed to a certain level of exposure. The use of an audible beeper has helped new radiology residents and other health workers gain an immediate awareness of radiation safety in clinical areas (Gray, 1979).

Patient Teaching

The government has joined in the effort to reduce the risks and cost of unnecessary x-rays. The U.S. Department of Health and Human Services will send a free x-ray and vaccination card on request.[2] This x-ray record card is wallet-size and can be carried to the physician, clinic, or hospital. The card should be filled in each time an x-ray is taken, including the date, type of exam, address where the x-rays are kept, and the name of the referring physician. Other tips for the public from Health and Human Services (1978) are:

1. Don't decide on your own that you need an x-ray.
2. Don't insist on an x-ray.
3. If your doctor orders an x-ray, ask how it will help with the diagnosis.
4. Tell your doctor about any similar x-rays you have had.
5. Ask if gonad shielding can be used for you and your children. (A lead apron should be routinely provided.)
6. Tell your doctor if you think you are pregnant.

---

[2]To get this free card write for 6516 to the Consumer Information Center, Pueblo, Colorado 81009.

Pregnant and Potentially Pregnant Women: The 14-Day Rule

Ideally, a woman in her childbearing years should only be x-rayed during her menses or 10 to 14 days after onset, to avoid any exposure to a fetus. The routine use of lead aprons will offer some protection to the fetus of the woman who is unaware that she is pregnant. The NCRP Report 54 (1979) gives guidelines to help the clinician schedule or postpone *elective* x-ray exams of the pregnant or potentially pregnant woman. This report also notes that the original recommendation was that women who might be pregnant should be x-rayed only up to 10 days after onset of menses (10-day rule). However, later recommendations changed the rule to up to 14 days after onset of menses (14-day rule). The 14-day rule is a tentative recommendation from the NCRP. A few hospitals have formal procedures about scheduling in relation to menses. Thus, nurses working with clients in the childbearing years should be aware of the 14-day rule for x-rays.

Benefit Versus Risk

Only recently has the public become aware of the health risks of unnecessary x-rays. Certainly the controversy about nuclear plants has caused an increased awareness by the public of the potential dangers from radiation. In addition to the potential health hazards from overuse of x-rays, the cost of unnecessary x-rays should also be considered. The cost of x-rays may be paid by insurance companies, but the cost is ultimately passed on to the consumer (Hales, 1980). If consumers can take more responsibility for avoiding unnecessary x-rays, there may be a financial gain as well as a decreased risk of illness or mutations from radiation exposure.

The point does need to be emphasized that if the patient needs an x-ray for diagnostic purposes, the benefit will far outweigh the risk. It is beyond the scope of nursing practice to evaluate the usefulness and safety of specific tests ordered for a patient. If the nurse encounters a patient who is refusing an x-ray because of a fear of radiation, it would probably be better to have the radiologist or physician explain the benefits of the test in comparison to any small risk of radiation. An informed public can cooperate with health professionals to reduce the possible risks and increased costs from x-ray tests. When x-rays are done, the patient should feel confident that the benefit of a specific test far outweighs the risk. The nurse can be instrumental in educating the public to have a healthy respect for x-rays as diagnostic tools.

PRETEST NURSING IMPLICATIONS

Clarifying Information about the Test

When radiology tests are necessary for a patient, the physician is responsible for informing the patient why the tests are needed and the benefits and risks associated with the specific tests. If an x-ray is part of an invasive test, a special permit will have to be signed. (See Chapter 6.) Most radiology departments have printed material that gives information about how the test is done and what is necessary for patient preparation. The role of the nurse is primarily to clarify the information the patient has received and follow up on anything that seems unclear. If there are no printed instructions or if the patient is unable to read, the nurse will have to explain the information. If the patient does not speak

English, an interpreter will be needed. The nurse must understand enough about the test to be able to give simple, accurate information to the patient. (Key points about specific tests are covered later in this chapter.)

Focusing on Sensation Information

Often the patient may be more concerned about what the test ''feels like'' than a technical explanation of the test itself. Hartfield (1981) studied the effects of procedural information, sensation information, and no information on the anxiety levels of patients having barium enemas. Patients who received sensation information reported less anxiety than the other groups. Nursing research for the past several years has suggested patients cope better with discomfort and pain if they are told what sensations to expect (Johnson, 1974).

Based on nursing research about preparing patients for painful procedures, McHugh et al. (1982) have suggested several guidelines:

- Physical sensations should be described, but not evaluated.
- Patients should be told what causes the sensations, (i.e., dye causes flushing) so they will not conclude something has gone wrong.
- Patients should be prepared for those aspects of the experience that are noticed by the majority of patients.

Specific questions about the interpretation of the test should be referred to the physician who is diagnosing the problem.

Relieving Anxiety

The nurse can often relieve much of the patient's anxiety by making sure that the patient has received all the information he or she needs about the test, including any preparations that are needed. However, even with adequate information many patients are anxious about x-rays. In addition to the fear of pain and discomfort from some x-rays, there is often a certain amount of worry about what might be found. The nurse must not overlook the psychological needs of the patient when focusing on the physical preparation. Patients may be relieved to find a nurse who not only listens but actively encourages them to ventilate any feelings they have about the upcoming test.

Promoting Patient Comfort

A study done in an English hospital identified four major factors that patients identified as being stressful during barium x-ray studies (Barnett, 1978): 1) waiting time in the x-ray department, 2) moving about on the hard x-ray table, 3) darkness and noise during the screening, and 4) enemas or suppositories that made the patients sleepless and exhausted before the test. An awareness of the physical factors likely to cause stress during x-ray studies should help the nurse plan care that is nurturing and supportive both before and after what many patients may experience as an ordeal.

The waiting time in the x-ray department may be very exhausting to some patients. The nurse can alert the x-ray department's personnel that the patient is confused or incontinent or in a great deal of pain so that the patient with a major problem is not left waiting for a long time. If a very weak patient must wait, a stretcher should be used for transportation rather than a wheelchair. If permissible, pain medication may be given before the trip. Because a number of x-ray tests require lying or moving about on a hard table, the patient should be well-rested. Enemas or suppositories should be done early enough so that the patient can rest awhile before going to x-ray. If possible, any exhausting treatments should be postponed until the patient returns from x-ray. If possible, the nurse can promise to let the patient rest once the x-ray is finished. For some patients, the waiting time in x-ray causes boredom. The nurse can encourage the patient to take some reading material or other activity, such as knitting, to help pass the time.

The nurse should see if the patient is ready for x-ray. Glasses, dentures, and hearing aides should not be removed before the x-ray if needed. X-ray personnel should be informed that a patient is hard of hearing or has other communication problems. The patient needs to empty his bladder. A robe should be worn for privacy and warmth, as well as slippers if the patient is to stand during the test.

These suggestions for ensuring patient comfort are basic and thus often not mentioned. However, unless the nurse attends to these details, the x-ray experience may be more uncomfortable than necessary. If the x-ray is being done on an out-patient basis, the nurse can give the patient tips on how to come prepared for x-ray. It is also important the patient know the approximate time for the x-rays so business or home affairs do not present problems.

Keeping the Patient NPO

The nurse must make sure that the patient understands when he or she is not allowed to eat or drink before a test (n.p.o.) With some tests, a light breakfast or clear liquid may be allowed. Patients may need clarification that clear liquids means just that. Orange juice, milk, and so on are not clear liquids—one cannot see through them. Because of dehydration, especially in the very young or the elderly, the nurse must find out if the test requires strict n.p.o. or if clear liquids are permissible. Most hospitals put an n.p.o. sign in the Kardex and on the door, but a well-informed patient is the best guarantee that the patient will observe n.p.o. status, if necessary. For children the restrictions on n.p.o. status may only be for three hours rather than the usual six to eight hours for adults.

Assessing the Effectiveness of Bowel Preparations

X-ray studies that involve structures in the lower abdomen may require a "bowel prep" before the x-ray. The preparation may be accomplished by cleansing enemas, cathartics, or suppositories. For example, a patient may be given a bisacodyl tablet (Dulcolax) or castor oil the night before the x-ray and a suppository the next morning. It is very important for the nurse to assess the effectiveness of the bowel preparation. If the method used did not cause an evacuation of the bowel, other methods may be needed before the patient is sent to x-ray. A poorly prepared patient may mean that the x-rays have to be repeated.

Children and Elderly. A series of cleansing enemas or strong cathartics or repeated suppositories may be very taxing to elderly, frail patients. The nurse should question "standard" orders for strong laxatives when the patient is very small or frail. Perhaps smaller doses will be sufficient. Cathartics or enemas may be contraindicated if the patient

TABLE 1. SUMMARY OF CRITERIA NEEDED FOR BOWEL PREPARATION[a]

1. Restriction of diet to clear liquids (check for times)
2. Hydration of the patient by adequate clear liquids (check for amounts)
3. Use of an evacuant that stimulates the small intestine (check for laxative ordered)
4. Use of an evacuant that stimulates the colon (check for laxatives or suppositories ordered)
5. Use of an enema as an additional cleansing method (check for orders for tap water enemas or small medicated enemas)

[a] *See text for more details on specific preps for various procedures.*

has had severe diarrhea or bleeding. Children under one-year old are usually not given any suppositories as bowel preparations. Children ages one to nine may be given a half suppository. Any dose of laxative must be calculated on the basis of the weight of the child.

Teaching at Home. When bowel preps are to be done in the home, the patient must be taught exactly what to do if the procedure does not clean out the bowel. Also, the patient needs to be shown exactly how to insert the suppository. Suppositories are always unwrapped before insertion. Often what is ''obvious'' to the health professional may not be to the patient. See Table 1 for a summary of the criteria needed to maximize bowel preparation.

Dyes Used as Contrast Media

Many of the dyes used as contrast media contain iodinated compounds, which have the potential to provoke allergic reactions (see Table 2). The radiology department should be notified if the patient has any allergies to iodine substances. The nurse should ask the patient if he or she has any allergies. For example, an allergy to seafood may be due to an allergy to iodine.

TABLE 2. NURSING IMPLICATIONS WHEN CONTRAST MEDIUM OR DYE IS USED FOR X-RAY TESTS

Examples of Common Radiologic Tests Using Iodine Contrast Medium or Dye
1. Gallbladder series (oral tablets)
2. Intravenous cholangiograms (IVC)
3. Intravenous pyelograms (IVP)
4. Arteriograms

Key Nursing Implications

Pretest[a]	*Posttest*
a. Assess for allergy to iodine	a. Assess for any allergic reactions
b. Instruct on sensations of dye	b. Encourage fluids
	c. Do not use urine for tests, specific gravity, etc., for 24 hours
	d. Assess for phlebitis at injection site

[a] *See text for details.*

Except for the oral tablets used for a gallbladder series, all administration of dyes are done in the radiology department. Before the radiologist injects the dye intravenously, the patient will again be questioned about possible allergies. Many of the dyes have an antihistamine in the preparation, but the radiologist still watches carefully for any signs of allergy, such as nausea, vomiting, palpitations, dyspnea, and dizziness. Radiology departments are always equipped with drugs (epinephrine, antihistamines, and corticosteroids) and equipment to treat anaphylactic shock, which can result from the dye.

Patients need to understand that normally the dye causes a flushed warm sensation when it is injected intravenously. The dye may also cause a salty taste in the mouth. Some references suggest to use the term "contrast medium" rather than "dye" when explaining tests to the patient. The word "dye" may give the impression that the material permanently changes body color, which it does not. The after-effects of the dye are covered in the next section. The section on diagnostic products in the Physician's Desk Reference (1982) gives detailed information on all the common contrast media used in x-ray exams.

POSTTEST NURSING IMPLICATIONS

The nurse needs to know exactly what type of procedure was done because specific implications are related to specific tests. (Care after a test is detailed under the description of the test later in this chapter.) Some hospitals may have a mini recovery room for patients who need special observation, such as neurologic checks (Maphet, 1981). More commonly, patients are returned to their rooms as soon as the procedures are finished.

Assessments for Reactions to Contrast Media

Usually if the patient is allergic to the dye, or contrast medium, an immediate allergic reaction will occur in the radiology department, but delayed reactions are possible; consequently, any symptoms such as urticaria, nausea, vomiting, or dyspnea should be reported immediately. Oral antihistamines or corticosteroids may be ordered for allergic reactions not acute enough to require epinephrine. Occasionally, the vein used for the dye injection may become inflammed. Any local tissue reactions should be reported. Warm compresses may be used for the phlebitis.

Dyes given intravenously for x-ray diagnostic tests are excreted in the urine. The dye acts as an osmotic diuretic. Thus, if other conditions permit, the patient who has a dye injection should be given extra fluid to replace the fluid lost with the excretion of the dye. Some patients may complain of some bladder irritation or burning on urination caused by the dye. The dye is not visible in the urine but it does elevate the specific gravity of the urine. (Note dye does not change the osmolality of the urine so a urine osmolality test would be a valid test of fluid balance. See Corbett, 1982.)

The contrast medium of barium sulfate, used for studies of the gastrointestinal tract, may cause constipation so fluids need to be encouraged after these x-rays. The barium is visible in the stool as white streaks.

Resuming Food Intake and Preventing Dehydration

The patient may be returned to the unit to wait until a second series of x-rays are taken. Usually the x-ray technician indicates that the patient is not yet finished or makes an appropriate note on the patient's chart. The nurse must make sure that the test is indeed completed and that food or water will not interfere with any follow-up x-rays. The patient may be very hungry or thirsty from being on n.p.o. status for a long time. If allowed and tolerated, a cup of tea or some milk will be most appreciated until more solid food can be obtained from the kitchen. The liquids can help eliminate the dehydration, which may develop from the extended n.p.o. status.

For many people, food is more than just physically satisfying. Food can be a symbol of love and care. Concern about the patient's lack of food may be interpreted by the patient as a very tangible sign of warmth and caring. (One of the cornerstones of professional nursing is nurturing.) It becomes very routine for the nurse to withhold food and fluids because of diagnostic procedures. It is not routine for the patient to go without food or fluids, and mere acknowledgment of this deprivation may be satisfying to the patient.

Providing Comfort and Pain Relief

Waiting in the radiology department and the test procedures themselves may be exhausting. Patients should, therefore, be allowed to rest and only be disturbed for necessary procedures, such as checking vital signs, inspecting dressings for bleeding, etc. Lying on a hard table will cause a backache for some people. A backrub will often be appreciated. A heating pad may also be helpful if muscles or joints hurt from the positioning during the test. (A physician's order is needed for heat applications.) Some procedures cause pain severe enough to require the use of analgesics. The nurse must assess whether the pain is the expected type for the procedure. For example, pain at the site of an arterial puncture would be expected, while pain in the foot may be a symptom of an embolus from the puncture site.

Special Needs of Outpatients

After diagnostic tests, an outpatient may need to rest before going home. If advisable, patients should be told in advance to have someone available to drive them home. The patient should be informed about the level of pain to be expected. For example, hystosalpingogram may cause severe abdominal pains a few hours after the procedure. The patient should be alerted that if the pain is not relieved by analgesics, she should notify the clinic or physician because pain can be a sign of a complication, such as a perforation. Arthrograms are another type of x-ray often done on an outpatient basis. The manipulation of the joint entailed in the procedure can cause severe pain. The patient may need to rest a while until he or she can walk out of the clinic or office. Instruction on the use of warm compresses or sitz baths to relax the tense, tired muscles from the painful x-ray session may be helpful.

Reducing Anxiety after Tests are Completed

Interpretation of the test results is usually not ready until the next day. The patient may be concerned about the results of the test. The nurse can act as a sounding board and help the patient formulate questions to ask the physician. The nurse can also let the patient vent feelings about any pain or discomfort experienced during the test.

IMPLICATIONS FOR FUTURE CARE

By listening to the patient's personal account of the test, the nurse not only helps the patient put the experience in perspective but learns something that might help in preparing the next patient for a radiologic test. As noted earlier, patients should be prepared for sensations experienced by the majority of patients undergoing a specific diagnostic procedure. McHugh (1982) suggests that nurses make lists of all aspects of a patient's experience. Then using the list, the nurse can interview patients to discover what aspects of the experience are noticed by at least 50 percent of the patients. The nurse will also discover what words are most often used to describe the sensations. Patients' descriptions are usually less technical and complex than nurses'.

SPECIFIC RADIOLOGIC TESTS

CHEST X-RAYS

Description: Chest x-rays are not only done in the radiology department but also at the patient's bedside, if the patient cannot be transported to the radiology department. However, bedside, portable chest x-rays are not of as good a quality as those in the radiology department. In the radiology department, the patient stands six to nine feet from the x-ray machine; whereas, the smaller, portable chest x-ray must be at most three feet from the patient. In the x-ray department, the standard chest film is a posterior–anterior (PA) view because the patient stands with the anterior part of the body next to the film. The portable chest x-ray only gives an anterior–posterior (AP) view because the film is behind the patient's back. In describing positions of the patient, the first term refers to the site of entry and the second term to the exit of the x-ray beam, which is captured on the film. Note the basic working principle: the part that needs to be studied should be next to the film (French, 1980). Chest x-rays may be lateral views or oblique views as well. If there is a question of free pleural fluid, the film is taken with the patient supine or in a lateral decubitus position, so that the fluid will pool. (Decubitus means a lying-down position; hence, a decubitus ulcer results from a lying-down position.) If air is suspected, the patient is kept sitting up. For most chest films, the patient is asked to take a deep breath and hold it so that the lungs are fully expanded and the diaphragm is descended.

Purposes: X-ray films of the chest are used to identify various abnormalities of the lungs and structures in the thorax. In addition, the size of the heart and abnormalities in the ribs or diaphragm can be determined. The three most common abnormalities seen in chest films are pneumonia, atelectasis, and pneumothorax (Tinker, 1976). Unfortunately, in early stages of tuberculosis or asthma the patient may have a normal chest x-ray. Also in chronic obstructive lung disease the chest x-ray may not correlate with the clinical status. Expiration films are used to detect a small pneumothorax or to demonstrate alterations in ventilation due to emphysema or partial bronchial obstructions (Wilson, 1977). Tumors of the lung can be identified by chest x-rays, but tomograms may give more information about the exact location in the tissue. (See tomograms in the next chapter.) As discussed earlier, chest x-rays are not done as routinely as they were because of the concern about too much radiation exposure.

Patient Preparation

A chest x-ray done in the radiology department requires no special preparation. The patient should not wear jewelry or any metal around the neck or on the hospital gown. Most patients are very familiar with the chest x-ray and realize that there is no pain or discomfort.

Nurse's Role with Portable Chest X-Rays

If a portable chest x-ray is used at the patient's bedside, the nurse may have a more active role in preparing the patient. For example, chest electrodes need to be temporarily removed so the metal will not interfere with the picture. Intravenous tubing, arterial lines, etc. may cause shadows; thus, nothing should be lying on top of the patient's chest. The patient's back needs to be in even contact with the film holder. If the patient is slumped in bed, the picture may be of very poor quality. Sometimes the nurse may be asked to hold the patient during the x-ray. If it is absolutely necessary for someone to help hold the patient in a position, the helper should wear a lead apron. (Lead gloves may also be used for protection.) As discussed earlier, although the radiation from one chest x-ray is minimal, the nurse must remember that radiation exposure is cumulative over a lifetime. Pregnant nurses should definitely not be exposed to any x-rays being done on patients. Nurses who could be pregnant should follow the 14-day rule discussed earlier (i.e., radiation only up to 14 days after onset of menses).

Posttest Nursing Implications

There are no special implications for nursing care after a chest x-ray. If the x-ray film shows atelectasis, the patient will need vigorous pulmonary toilet.

PLAIN FILMS OF THE ABDOMEN: FLAT PLATES, THREE-WAY FILMS, AND KUB

Description: Plain films, or scout films, of the abdomen may be done as the first step in assessing a variety of abdominal problems. They may be used with the patient lying down flat, turned to the left, and upright. These three positions are called a three-way abdominal x-ray. If the main focus is on the *k*idneys, *u*reters, and *b*ladders, the x-ray is called a KUB.

Purposes: Abdominal x-rays can detect loops of dilated bowel, patterns of gas, and possible obstructions. Stones and calcified areas in the pancreas, biliary system, or urinary system may be detected but films with contrast medium are needed for diagnosis.

Perforations in the gastrointestinal tract will result in the escape of air into the peritoneal cavity, which will cause an elevation of the diaphragm on the affected side. The elevated diaphragm will be seen on the plain film.

Patient Preparation

In abdominal trauma, the flat plate x-ray will be ordered as a stat procedure. If there are questionable abdominal injuries, there will not be any attempt to clear the bowel of feces and gas. In nontraumatic conditions, however, the patient may need a bowel preparation before the x-ray is done. (See the introductory remarks on types of bowel preparation that may be done.)

Nursing Implications

There are no special nursing implications related to a flat plate x-ray of the abdomen. However, the nurse should be aware that the patient may be scheduled for other x-rays that involve the use of a contrast medium to identify particular structures. The nurse should also assess and record the exact nature of any abdominal pain; this could be useful in the differential diagnosis of acute abdominal problems.

BONE OR SKELETAL X-RAYS, INCLUDING THE SKULL

Description and Purpose: Skeletal x-rays are routinely used to detect fractures. They may also be used to detect tumors of the bone, but scans are more useful. (See Chapter 3 for the use of bone scans with radionuclides to detect tumors.) Simple x-rays are useful in assessing skull fractures; however, the presence or absence of a skull fracture does not correlate with the possible severity of any underlying brain damage. (The CT scan discussed in the next chapter is extremely valuable in detecting soft tissue injuries.) Skeletal x-rays are also used to assess arthritic conditions and to detect osteomyletitis.

Patient Preparation

Skeletal x-rays require no special preparation. If the x-rays are being done to assess a possible fracture, the patient should be treated as having a fracture until it is ruled out. The patient needs careful handling and immobilization of the affected part. Pain relief may be needed before transportation. If skull x-rays are required, the patient should have a neurologic assessment before transportation to the radiology department. The nurse should notify the members of the x-ray department of any instability in the patient's vital signs, so that the x-rays are done immediately and the patient watched carefully.

Nursing Implications

See the precautions noted in the preparation before bone films regarding care of potential fractures. If the patient is having skeletal x-rays because of arthritis, the patient may need warmth to the joints and some analgesic after the manipulation.

UPPER GI SERIES, CARDIAC SERIES, AND SMALL BOWEL SERIES

Description and Purposes: Barium swallows are used for x-rays of the upper gastrointestinal (GI) tract and to outline the cardiac border. The patient drinks barium sulfate, which is a chalky radiopaque substance. Its nonwater soluble quality prevents it from being absorbed by the gastrointestinal tract. If there is a possibility of a leak or an obstruction, the radiologist will use a dye, meglucamine diatrizoate (Gastrograffin), which is water soluble. Fluoroscopy during the barium swallow will outline the esophagus and any structural defects. If the barium swallow is being done to outline the borders of the heart, the size and contour of the heart will be revealed. Several different views of the heart can be photographed, called a "cardiac series." Esophageal varices may also show on the film.

The swallowed barium coats the stomach walls so that defects, such as tumors or ulcers, are seen as dark areas with a white background of the dye. The upper GI series is the definitive test for stomach and duodenal ulcers. The time it takes for the barium to empty out of the stomach will be important in some cases because duodenal ulcers may cause some degree of pyloric obstruction or gastric outlet obstruction. As the barium goes through the small intestine another series of x-rays may be taken, called a small bowel series.

An upper GI series takes about 45 minutes. If a small bowel series is done, it may take up to five hours to complete the x-rays. Also, a follow-up x-ray may be taken in 24 hours.

Certain drugs may be given during an upper GI series. For example, glucagon may be given to relax the bowel. Drugs may also be used to accelerate the passage of barium through the stomach and small bowel to promote better visualization of the jejunum and ileum. Metoclopromide (Reglan by Robbins) is such a promotility agent. These drugs are given intravenously after the patient is in x-ray.

Patient Preparation

The patient usually has a light diet the evening before the x-ray and has n.p.o. status from midnight until the test. Food or medicine in the gastrointestinal tract will interfere with the barium coating the walls. Sometimes oral medications may be continued until two hours prior to the scheduled exam, if gastric emptying is normal. However, any administration of medications should be cleared by the physician. Some parenteral medications, such as antibiotics, are continued; others may not be, for example, regular insulin would be withheld while a longer acting insulin may be given. Because narcotics and anticholinergic drugs, such as atropine, slow down the mobility of the intestinal tract, the radiologist should be notified if these drugs have been given to the patient. Sometimes atropine might be ordered before an upper GI series if the patient has a hyperactive bowel. The patient should be told that fluoroscopy is done in the dark and that the x-ray table is tilted to help the flow of barium. If a small bowel series is to be done, the patient needs to know that it is a lengthy procedure requiring a couple of trips to the x-ray department. The patient should also be told that the barium has a chalky taste. Many radiology departments use flavored barium sulfate (e.g., peppermint or chocolate), but most patients still find it rather unpleasant to drink.

Posttest Nursing Implications

The patient may be returned to the unit to wait for a second series of x-rays to be taken. Food and water should not be allowed until the radiologist completes the test. If the patient has an ulcer, the lack of food in the stomach may have aggravated the abdominal pain, so food or antacids should be resumed as soon as possible. The patient should be informed that his or her stool will be light-colored due to the barium being excreted. For some patients, the barium may be constipating. Thus, the nurse should note that the patient is well-hydrated, that there is adequate roughage in his or her diet. Laxatives or enemas may be needed. Barium in the intestine will interfere with other abdominal tests, so they should be scheduled first; otherwise, the patient may need an enema so that other structures can be visualized by these other tests.

BARIUM ENEMAS

Description: For examination of the lower colon an enema of barium sulfate is given. This is done in the radiology department. The patient must retain the barium while a series of x-ray pictures are taken. After the barium is excreted a final x-ray of the bowel is taken. Sometimes air is put into the empty colon afterwards for a double contrast exam. The introduction of air may cause slight discomfort. A barium enema takes about an hour or hour-and-a-half to complete.

Purpose: The barium enema is commonly used for any kind of suspected lower intestine or colon problem. Tumors, strictures, polyps, and diverticulum can all be well visualized by this method. Sometimes the barium enema is also therapeutic; it may reduce an obstruction if caused by intussusception or telescoping of the bowel.

Patient Preparation

The lower colon must be prepared by the bowel preparation used in a particular setting. As mentioned in the general implications, bowel preps may include enemas, laxative, or suppositories. It is essential that there not be any fecal matter in the lower colon. The patient may be given a cleansing enema early the morning of the x-ray. Some institutions do not schedule enemas the day of the x-ray. If the patient has a severely inflammed bowel or active bleeding, strong cathartics or other bowel preps are contraindicated.

Restriction of Food

A liquid diet may be ordered for the day before the exam. Patients are given a light breakfast the day of the exam because the food will not reach the large intestine by the time of the exam. However, if there is any question about complications, food may be withheld. Perforation of the colon is a very unlikely complication, but it can occur if the bowel is diseased and friable. In the case where there may be complications, it is always better that the patient not have a full stomach. Adequate ingestion of liquids is important so that the patient is well-hydrated. An example of patient instructions for use with outpatients is shown in Table 3.

If the patient is unable to retain the fluid of the enema, the nurse needs to inform the radiology department so a special tube can be used to instill the contrast medium. The

TABLE 3. INSTRUCTIONS FOR BARIUM ENEMA

THE SENOKOT SUPPOSITORY AND X-PREP LIQUID MUST BE PURCHASED AT THE PHARMACY. (*Senokot* and *X-prep* are brand names for senna preparations)—biscoday 1 (*Dulcolax*) may also be used.)

ON THE DAY BEFORE YOUR APPOINTMENT—EAT AND DRINK ONLY THE FOLLOWING:

LUNCH This meal may include clear broth, white chicken meat sandwich (no butter, lettuce or other additive), or two hard boiled eggs, strained fruit juices, jello or gelatine (not including fruits or nuts), coffee or tea (without cream or milk), or carbonated beverages.

3 P.M. Take 2½ oz. of the prescribed laxative and drink one full glass of water.

SUPPER Limit your evening meal to liquids without milk products. This meal may include clear broth, strained fruit juices, jello or gelatine (not containing fruits or nuts), coffee or tea (without cream or milk), or carbonated beverages.

10 P.M. Insert one unwrapped *Senokot* or other suppository into your rectum.

ON THE DAY OF YOUR APPOINTMENT:

BREAKFAST Limit to coffee or tea (without cream or milk), strained fruit juices, dry toast or bread.

Two (2) hours before your scheduled examination, insert one unwrapped *Senokot* or other suppository into your rectum.

PLEASE REPORT TO THE X-RAY DEPARTMENT ON ______________ AT _____

WHAT IS THE BARIUM ENEMA?

This is the x-ray examination of the large intestine. For this study it is most important to clean the bowel of all retained fecal matter. A tube will be placed into your rectum, and the barium liquid will flow easily into your bowel. The radiologist will study the bowel under the fluoroscope, and have several x-rays taken.

NOTE: If you have severe diarrhea or considerable rectal bleeding, consult your physician before taking the laxative or suppository requested above. If you have any questions, or require a change of appointment, please call the x-ray department.

Courtesy of Kaiser Permanente Medical Group, San Francisco, California.

patient who can retain the enema fluid can be spared this extra discomfort. Most people can retain the amount of fluid used for the barium enema, but it is often a concern for the patient.

A barium enema can be administered through a colostomy. Usual bowel preparations are done that would include irrigation of the colostomy before the procedure. Arnell & Nassberg (1981) describe, in detail, the techniques used to instill barium via a colostomy.

Posttest Nursing Implications

A barium enema can be exhausting physically and psychologically. It is embarassing to many people to be given an enema in the radiology department and then to be asked to assume awkward positions in front of other people. If the patient did not retain the barium well, a bath may be in order. Although most patients do expel the barium in the x-ray department, some, particularly the elderly, may become constipated from barium still in the intestines. Fluids should be encouraged, 2000 ml a day for the adult, unless contraindicated. Cleansing enemas or laxative may be given if there is a problem with defecation. If the barium was instilled via a colostomy, irrigations can rid the bowel of the residual barium. As mentioned earlier, the patient's first stool will be a light color or will have white streaks.

ORAL CHOLECYSTOGRAM OR GALLBLADDER SERIES

Description: For an oral cholecystogram (OCG), six dye tablets are taken orally the night before the x-ray. The tablets contain iodinated compounds, such as iopanioc acid (Telpaque), iodoalphionic acid (Priodox), or sodium ipodate (Oragrafin). The radiopaque dye or contrast medium is excreted via the liver into the biliary system and concentrates in the gallbladder. Dye is not given if the patient has any liver dysfunction. For example, a bilirubin above 3 or 4 mgl/dl would be a contraindication for a gallbladder (GB) series.
Purposes: The GB series is used to determine if a gallbladder can fill, concentrate, and empty bile properly. The presence of stones will be seen as light shadows in the gallbladder. If the gallbladder is not visualized on the x-ray film, the test may be repeated with a double dose (12 tablets) of dye. If the gallbladder is still not visualized, this may indicate an obstruction in the biliary tree or a diseased gallbladder. The patient may be given a fatty meal after the OCG and more films may be later taken to see how well the gallbladder empties. (Note that the use of ultrasound is a newer diagnostic test for gallstones, see Chapter 4, as is radionuclides, see Chapter 3.)

Patient Preparation

A low fat diet is given the evening before a GB series, so the gallbladder will not be stimulated to empty. Some radiology departments may start patient preparation two days before the exam. On the first evening, the patient is given a high-fat meal (milk, eggs, and bread with butter), followed by dye tablets. The next evening, a normal meal without fats is given, followed by a second dose of six tablets. This double dose of tablets may eliminate some cases of nonvisualization of the gallbladder, which are due to lack of dye and not gallbladder disease.

Because the oral tablets contain iodine, the patient must be checked for any sensitivity to iodine compounds. The six tablets are taken after the evening meal, one every five minutes with water. After the six tablets are taken, the patient is placed on n.p.o. status. The tablets may cause nausea, vomiting, and diarrhea in some patients. If the patient vomits the tablets, the test will have to be rescheduled. Diarrhea will not cause loss of the dye. If the patient cannot swallow the tablets, a contrast medium can be given intravenously in the radiology department. However, the intravenous cholangiograms are usually used to assess the condition of the ducts, not the concentrating ability of the gallbladder. (See the next section.) A bowel prep of enemas or suppositories may be ordered to clean out the bowel. If the patient has received morphine sulfate, the radiologist should be notified because morphine may cause spasm of the sphincter of Oddi.

Posttest Nursing Implications

As mentioned earlier, the patient may be given a fatty meal if more films are planned to see how well the gallbladder empties. Otherwise, the patient can resume whatever diet is tolerated. Actually, a fat-restricted diet is often needed because of the patient's fat intolerance due to an obstruction of the biliary system. (See a nursing text for a discussion about the nursing implications when a patient has an obstruction of the biliary system.)

CHOLANGIOGRAMS: INTRAVENOUS, OPERATIVE, TRANSHEPATIC, AND VIA ENDOSCOPE

Description and Purposes: A cholangiogram is an x-ray of the biliary tree using contrast medium so the cystic, hepatic, and common bile ducts can be visualized. Note that the oral cholecystogram, discussed above, is used to assess the ability of the gallbladder to concentrate and excrete the dye.

IVC. When the dye is given intravenously (IVC), the liver excretes the dye into the biliary tree. X-ray pictures are taken at intervals after the dye is injected, and begins to appear in the biliary tree about 10 minutes after the intravenous administration of the dye. It takes about four hours but sometimes eight hours for the dye to be totally excreted, so the patient may be in the radiology department for several hours.

Via T-Tubes. Cholangiograms are also done during surgical procedures to check for stones in the common bile duct, which might not be seen or felt. With the operative method, the dye is injected directly into a drainage catheter (T-tube), placed in the common bile duct during surgery. X-ray films are taken immediately after the dye is instilled. A cholangiogram via the T-tube may also be done several days postoperatively to evaluate the patency of the biliary tree. Patients with exploration of the common bile duct have T-tubes for bile drainage until the edema in the common bile duct is gone (Phipps, et al. 1979).

Transhepatic. Transhepatic cholangiograms are done via a percutaneous insertion of a needle into the common bile duct. It is done with the aid of fluoroscopy. After the needle is in the common bile duct, dye is injected.

Endoscopic. A fourth way to inject dye into the biliary system is with the use of an endoscope passed down the gastrointestinal tract through the sphincter of Oddi into the biliary tract. (See Chapter 8 for a discussion about endoscopic procedures.)

Patient Preparation

Of the four procedures described above, IVC is most commonly used. The patient is kept on n.p.o. status for six to eight hours before the test. A bowel preparation will be ordered to clear the intestinal tract. The IVC is done in the radiology department and is not particularly uncomfortable except for the sensation of dye being injected intravenously.

If cholangiograms are part of an operative procedure, the patient receives the routine preoperative preparation. A percutaneous transhepatic cholangiogram is done in the radiology department. Because this is an invasive procedure, the physician must explain the specific risks to the patient. The endoscopic procedure is also invasive and entails certain risks; consequently, institutions will have special protocols to follow regarding permission. (See Chapter 6 for nursing implications for invasive tests.) Because obstructions in the biliary system tend to increase bleeding, the patient usually has a prothrombin time done before any type of invasive procedure of the biliary tree. If the prothrombin time is increased, vitamin K must be given parenterally before traumatic tests are done. Gastrointestinal absorption of vitamin K, a fat soluble vitamin, is hampered when there is a biliary obstruction; there is a lack of bile salts for fat absorption. Corbett (1982) discusses laboratory tests used to assess for biliary obstruction and the nursing implications for patients with elevation of direct bilirubin (obstructive jaundice).

Posttest Nursing Implications

The after-care for the patient who has had dye instilled via an IVC would be the routine nursing discussed in the beginning of this chapter.

See Chapter 6 for the nursing implications when a patient has had an invasive procedure that may cause bleeding. Frequent checking of vital signs and bed rest for a certain amount of time is important. Just as in a liver biopsy, complications such as leakage of bile into the peritoneal cavity can occur when a needle is put into the common bile duct. Any abdominal pain, which could mean bile peritonitis, should be called to the attention of the physician. Chills and fever may be due to inflammation of the bile duct.

INTRAVENOUS PYELOGRAM

Description: Sodium diatrizoate (Hyopaque) or megalumine diatrizoate (Renografin) are dyes used for pyelograms because they are excreted by the urinary system. Another name for an intravenous pyelogram (IVP) is an excretory urography because it demonstrates the ability of the entire urinary tract to excrete dye. After the dye or contrast medium has been injected intravenously, x-ray films are taken every minute for five minutes, allowing visualization of the cortex of the kidney. Approximately 15 minutes later, x-ray films are taken as the dye collects in the pelvis of the kidney and is excreted via the ureters into the bladder. The dye outlines the bladder in about 45 minutes. The patient is asked to void, and a postvoiding film is taken to see how well the bladder empties. The entire set of x-rays takes about an hour.

Purposes: Structural defects or tumors can be observed when the urinary system is outlined with dye. A retrograde introduction of dye, through ureteral catheters, to outline the urinary system is done via a cystoscope. (See Chapter 8 for endoscope procedures.) Note that renograms done with radionuclides (Chapter 3) can be done if patients are allergic to the contrast medium used for IVP.

Patient Preparation

The patient is given a light meal the evening before the test. Different radiology departments may have different instructions regarding n.p.o. status. Some radiologists prefer that the patient not take in any fluids so the dye will not be diluted. Other radiologists want the patient to be given clear liquids so that the patient is not dehydrated before the exam. A lack of normal renal function may make it hazardous for the patient to receive dye that is excreted via the kidney; therefore, serum creatine and BUN levels are assessed before the test is begun. The bowel prep for an IVP needs to be thorough. A cathartic as well as suppositories the evening before and the morning of the exam may be necessary. Enemas may be necessary if the patient has had barium studies in the preceding 48 hours.

The patient should be instructed about the feeling of the dye being injected. (See the general implications about contrast medium discussed earlier in this chapter.) There may be more than one venipuncture. The only other discomfort will result from lying in one position during the series of films. Voiding in the x-ray department may be embarassing for patients who must use a urinal or bedpan if they cannot go to the bathroom.

Posttest Nursing Implications

See the general implications for dye use, including a fluid intake of 2000 to 3000 ml of fluids. The patient should be observed for any signs of urinary problems, such as difficulty voiding or bladder irritation. Note that the serum creatine levels and/or creatine clearance tests may be used to assess any loss of renal function.

BRONCHOGRAM

Description: A bronchogram is an x-ray picture of the bronchial tree, in conjunction with a bronchoscopy. (See Chapter 8 for the nursing implications when a patient has a bronchoscopy.) An iodine dye is instilled by an atomizer or other means into the bronchi. X-ray films are made to show the outline and structure of the bronchial tree and lungs.

ARTERIOGRAMS

Description: Angiogram is a broad term meaning visualization of vessels that are either arteries, veins, or lymph channels. *Arteriogram* is a more precise term designating visualization of an arterial vessel or vessels. The most common site of dye injection for an arteriogram is the femoral artery. Arterial catheters are positioned, using a guidewire to advance the catheter to a certain spot in the arterial tree. Because the arterial catheter is radiopaque, movement of the catheter is noted by fluoroscopy. After the correct placement is obtained, dye is injected into the catheter to outline a certain portion of the artery.

In this way the circulation in the lower extremity can be visualized. Also, the catheter can be threaded, via the femoral artery, into the abdominal aorta to the level of the renal arteries for renal arteriograms. The arteries of the gastrointestinal tract can be visualized if the dye is instilled in the celiac axis. The branchial artery can be used for upper extremity visualization. Cartoid arteriograms may also be done, but can disrupt athrosclerotic plaques, which can become cerebral emboli. Therefore, the cartoid arteries are usually visualized by a catheter threaded through other arteries.
Purposes: Arteriograms are extremely valuable for observing the blood flow to a part of the body and to detect lesions, which may be amenable to surgery. The catheter used to confirm the diagnosis of a suspected kidney or liver lesion may also become a vehicle for the selective delivery of chemotherapeutic drugs or drugs to stop bleeding. Some researchers are also using catheters in arteries to remove atherosclerotic plaques (Athanasoulis, 1980).

Patient Preparation

The patient must sign a special permit form. (See Chapter 6 for the nurse's role in preparing patients for invasive procedures.) Because this test involves the use of an iodinated dye intravenously, the implications for dye use should be considered. (See the discussion on dyes in the beginning of this chapter.) The patient is kept on n.p.o. status for six to eight hours before the procedure; some institutions do allow liquids before an arteriogram. There may be an order to shave an area, but usually any preparation of the puncture site is done in the radiology department.

Posttest Nursing Implications

The patient is kept on bedrest for a minimum of six hours, to decrease the possibility of bleeding from the puncture site; some institutions may keep the patient on bedrest for 24 hours. The nurse should make an observation of the puncture site as soon as the patient returns from the radiology department, which will serve as a baseline comparison if there is any later bleeding on the dressing or some swelling around the site. There may be more than one site if one puncture was not successful. The pressure dressing, on the site, should not be removed. An icebag may also be placed on the site to decrease the possibility of bleeding or hematoma formation. Vital signs should be taken every 15 minutes for the first hour and then every two to four hours as ordered or deemed necessary. Frequent temperature checks are not necessary, but should be noted every four hours, to detect a beginning septicema or a reaction to the dye. Pulses distal to the arterial puncture must also be checked along with the vital signs. Thromus formation, emboli release, nerve damage, or spasms of the artery are all possible complications. Pain at the puncture site is not uncommon and may require analgesics, but pain distal to the puncture site may indicate an embolism.

Femoral Arteriogram. For a *femoral* arteriogram the pedal pulses are checked. (See Chapter 4 for the use of the Doppler instrument to assess arterial pulses.) The patient may not have had detectable pulses before the arteriogram; this must be taken into account. The color, sensation, and warmth of the foot examined should be compared with the other foot. Any pain in the foot or leg should be carefully assessed and compared to the pain before the arteriogram.

Brachial Arteriogram. If a *brachial* arteriogram is done, there is concern not only for spasm, embolism, or thrombus formation but also nerve compression. Pain or numbness in the fingers or hand should always be reported immediately. Blood pressure readings should not be taken on the examined arm because they temporarily compromise arterial circulation in the lower arm.

Carotid Arteriogram. For a *carotid* arteriogram, both temporal pulses should be checked. In addition, the patient should be assessed for any signs of transient ischemis attacks (TIA), such as facial weakness, visual disturbances, or slurred speech. The patient's head should be kept elevated about 30 degrees. A light ice collar may be used to reduce swelling. Pressure on the carotid arterial site should be avoided, this can cause a vagal response that can slow the heart. Tracheal obstruction can result from swelling, so the patient should be observed for any difficulty in breathing or swallowing. A tracheostomy set should be near by.

Renal Arteriogram. If a *renal* arteriogram is done, hypotension may result from a decrease in the formation of renin for a short time (Tucker, 1980). Fortunately, all of these complications from arteriograms are rare occurrences, but the nurse who makes skilled assessments may detect a problem before it becomes major.

VENOGRAMS

Description: A dye or contrast medium can be injected into a vein by a venipuncture or by a cutdown to view the venous system of particular organs or to evaluate flow to a particular area, for example, x-ray films taken as the dye goes through the venous system of the leg. It may be injected into a catheter in the femoral vein or inferior vena cava, and the catheter can be threaded to various organs to inspect details in the venous supply of the organ. A right-sided cardiac catheterization, for example, uses a vein for dye instillation. *Purposes*: Venograms may be useful in detecting deep vein thrombosis (DVT) or to assess other venous abnormalities, such as congenital abnormalities or incompetent valves. Venograms only show structure and flow. Radioisotopes (see Chapter 3) are more useful to assess the function of a specific tissue.

Patient Preparation

See the guidelines for arteriograms. Also see Chapter 7 on right-sided cardiac catheterization.

Posttest Nursing Implications

There are no restrictions on eating. The patient is usually not confined to bedrest, as with an arteriogram. And there are fewer complications from venous puncture as compared to arterial puncture. However, the nurse should carefully assess vital signs and check for any signs of hematoma formation. Phlebitis may result and warm compresses can be used to ease the pain of an irritated vein. The implications for the use of a dye must be noted as discussed earlier in this chapter. If a cutdown was necessary, the area must be assessed for potential infection.

LYMPHOGRAMS

Description: Visualization of the lymph system can be achieved by an injection of dye or contrast medium into the lymph system of an arm or leg. A dye (Evans blue) is first injected into the web of skin between the first and second toes or between the fingers. The blue dye is picked up by the lymph system. After approximately 30 minutes the lymph system is outlined, and a lymph vessel is then dissected and a small catheter inserted for the injection of an iodine dye (Ethidol). X-ray films are taken after the iodine dye is injected and again 24 hours later. Other x-ray pictures may be taken later because the lymph nodes retain the contrast medium for several weeks, even months.
Purposes: Enlarged and diseased lymph nodes can be identified on the films. Also, the lymphogram can show not only the extent of the disease, such as a lymphoma or Hodgkin's disease, but also the effectiveness of therapy.

Patient Preparation

The patient may be kept on n.p.o. status or may be allowed to eat. The patient should be prepared for some discomfort when the hand or foot is given a local anesthetic. The hardest part of the procedure may be lying still for the extent of the procedure, which may be up to three hours.

Posttest Nursing Implications

To prevent edema, the patient should keep the affected limb elevated for 24 hours. Vital signs should be checked to detect any signs of bleeding, infection, or adverse reactions to the dye.

The site of the dissection may become painful as the local anesthetic wears off, and mild analgesics may be needed for the incisional pain. Any numbness in the extremity distal to the incision should be reported immediately because of possible nerve damage. The site will have a few stitches, which need to be removed in seven to ten days, that should not get wet for a day or two. The site should be examined for any sign of infection and warm compresses applied to ease any discomfort from inflammation. If dye travels to the lung, via the thoracic duct, the patient may develop pneumonia. Thus, respiratory problems should be evaluated by the physician. Skin discoloration from the blue dye will fade in a few days. Stool and urine will also show some discoloration.

HYSTEROSALPINGOGRAM

Description: The patient is placed in the lithotomy position, and a vaginal speculum is inserted. Dye (Ethidol or Salpix) is injected through the cervix into the uterus and Fallopian tubes. The patient is awake during the procedure. There is likely to be some abdominal discomfort from the pressure of the dye, even though only about 10 ml are used. The exam is scheduled within a week to 10 days after the patient's menstrual period, to ensure that the patient is not pregnant. The test takes about half an hour.
Purposes: The test is used to detect blocked Fallopian tubes. Other abnormalities in the uterus, such as fibroids, will also be demonstrated on the x-ray. This is one of the tests

done as part of an infertility work-up. (See Chapter 9 for a discussion on the five basic tests for infertility.) Occasionally, the injection of the dye may also be done to evaluate the success of a tubal ligation.

Patient Preparation

A hysterosalpingogram is often done on an outpatient basis. There are no restrictions of food or fluid. The patient should have finished a menstrual period within the preceding seven to ten days. The patient will need to void right before the procedure. Although some institutions have the patient take an enema or suppository before the exam, no special bowel prep is usually necessary. The patient must remove her clothes from the waist down. Some patients are given a mild sedative. (See Chapter 6 on ways nurses can help prepare patients to cope with painful procedures.)

Posttest Nursing Implications

A few hours after the procedure, the patient may have severe uterine cramps that require analgesia. Warm sitz baths may be soothing, too. Although rare, perforation of the uterus can occur, so any severe cramping or profuse bleeding should be called to the attention of the physician or clinic. The patient may have some vaginal spotting for a day or two so she should be informed about the possible need of sanitary napkins.

MAMMOGRAMS

Description: A mammogram is an x-ray of the breasts to detect the presence of tumors too small to be discovered by palpation. Mammograms may include the injection of a dye into the mammary ducts, but routine screening procedures do not include the use of a contrast medium. Dye is useful in identifying intraductal papillomas. During the x-ray, the patient lies or sits with breasts pushed against the film holder. An inflated rubber cushion is used to decrease the discomfort of the flattened breasts against the film holder. The procedure takes about 45 to 60 minutes to complete. It is usually done on an outpatient basis as a screening device for women susceptible to the development of breast cancer.

Purposes: Because breast cancer is the leading cause of cancer in women, mass screening for this disease is needed. Mammograms became popular in the early 1960s as a tool to detect early breast cancer (Gorringe, 1978). However, in the late 1970s, concern about radiation risks caused a reevaluation of whether mammograms should be done routinely. The latest recommendation of the American Cancer Society (February, 1980) is that women should have mammograms done once between the ages of 35 and 40 to establish a reference, and further testing before age 50 should be done on the advice of the individual physician. For example, women with fibrocystic disease or a family history of breast cancer are considered high-risk individuals and a physician may advise yearly mammograms. The American Cancer Society does recommend that mammograms be done once a year for women after the age 50. Xeromammography, which uses a special kind of aluminum plate, subjects the patient to less radiation exposure than mammograms done with conventional roentgen film.

Patient Preparation

The patient should not use deodorant, perfume, or powder on the day of the test; these chemicals may interfere with the x-ray picture. The patient should wear clothing easy to remove from the waist up. The patient should be prepared for some physical discomfort, related to the manipulation of tender tissue, particularly if the breasts are pendulous. Otherwise, the test is not physically painful, but it may be traumatic to be exposed. The potential diagnosis of cancer may also create much anxiety.

Posttest Nursing Implications

There are no specific nursing implications; however, the nurse should assess if the patient knows how to do a self-examination of the breast. (See Chapter 6 on breast biopsies for follow-up of lumps in the breast.)

MYELOGRAMS

Description: A myelogram is an x-ray film of the subarachnoid space of the spinal column, in which air or dye may be used as a contrast medium. The dye may either be an oily contrast or a water soluble medium. If an oil-based dye is used, it is removed at the end of the procedure. The water-soluble dye is not. The dye or air is injected via a lumbar puncture. The patient will be on a tilted table to allow the dye flow to different parts of the spinal column.

Purposes: X-ray films, taken after the contrast medium is instilled, can show distortions of the spinal cord due to tumors or changes in the bone structures. Herniations or protrusions of intervertebral discs can also be visualized. (Note that the use of the computerized axial tomography (CT scanning) may eventually replace this test; see the next chapter.)

Patient Preparation

The patient's allergy history is important if iodine dye is being used. He or she should be on n.p.o. status for four to six hours, and a bowel prep may be ordered. The patient should be prepared for the positioning necessary for a lumbar puncture. (See Chapter 6 on lumbar punctures.) Sedatives may be ordered. Consent forms are needed.

Posttest Nursing Implications

If dye is used, the patient should be kept flat in bed for six to eight hours after it is removed. Some situations may require 24 hours of bedrest, depending on the type of dye (Maphet, 1981), but the patient can be turned from side to side. If the water-soluble dye was not removed, the head should be kept slightly elevated to keep the dye from irritating the cerebral meninges. The patient may need analgesics if headache, pain, and stiffness in the neck occur. If conditions permit, fluids should be encouraged to at least 2000 ml for the adult, to help with the production of adequate cerebral spinal fluid. The motor and sensations of the lower extremities should be assessed to make sure there was no nerve damage. The voiding pattern of the patient should be assessed to detect any urinary problems.

PNEUMOENCEPHALOGRAMS AND VENTRICULOGRAMS

Description: A pneumoencephalogram (PEG) is an x-ray film of the ventricles and meningeal spaces in the brain after air, oxygen, or helium is inserted into the subarachnoid spaces. The use of gas as a contrast medium makes it possible to identify space-occupying lesions in the brain. For a ventriculogram, air is injected directly into the ventricles through burr holes in the skull. Both of these neurologic procedures require special equipment, and are thus often done in a special operative suite.
Purposes: These are older tests used to detect tumors or other space-occupying lesions in the brain. The use of the CT scan has reduced dramatically the need to do pneumoencephalograms and ventriculograms. (The CT scan is covered in the next chapter.) Also, the use of ultrasound encephalograms (see Chapter 4) are making these tests obsolete.

Patient Preparation

The patient is usually prepared much as for neurologic surgery: n.p.o. status is maintained, consent forms signed, and sedation given. The patient should void. He or she remains awake during the procedure. Meticulous neurologic assessment is required of the nurse, who is present during these procedures.

Posttest Nursing Implications

Headaches are common, and ice bags may be used to provide some relief. Mild analgesics may be prescribed, but narcotics may be dangerous if there is any potential change in the patient's level of consciousness. The patient can be turned from side to side to hasten the absorption of the air. He or she should be watched for any signs of increasing intracranial pressure or shock. Taylor (1980) detailed nursing care for the patient having complex neurologic diagnostic work-ups.

Questions

1. A radiologic test where the patient is put in front of an x-ray tube and a screen is held over the part to be examined so that movement can be visualized is called a

a. Tomogram
b. Fluoroscopic examination
c. Laminagram or planinagram
d. CT scan

2. Which of these densities allows the most penetration of x-rays, and thus show up the blackest on x-ray film?

a. Fat tissue
b. Air
c. Bone
d. Water

3. The three methods to provide radiation protection when x-rays are used as diagnostic procedures include all the following *except*

   a. Scheduling x-rays a few days apart so there is a time interval between exposures
   b. Shielding the patient with lead aprons to protect uninvolved areas
   c. Having all personnel maintain distance when the x-ray machine is in use
   d. Making the exposure for the patient as short as possible

4. The American Cancer Society's recommendation (February 1980) for the use of the chest x-ray to detect lung cancer is that the annual chest x-ray should

   a. Be eliminated
   b. Be done only for smokers
   c. Be done for people over 50
   d. Continue to be part of an annual check-up

5. The American Cancer Society's recommendation (February, 1980) for the use of mammograms as screening devices for breast cancer is that all women have *annual* mammograms after age

   a. 35
   b. 40
   c. 45
   d. 50

6. All of the following are ways for consumers to protect themselves from unnecessary x-ray exposure *except*

   a. Asking for a lead apron to be used if dental x-rays are needed
   b. Carrying a card that lists all the x-rays that have been done of the person
   c. Asking the physician to explain how x-rays will help with the diagnosis
   d. Requesting x-rays to validate any unexplained symptoms

7. Factors that patients have identified as being stressful for barium x-ray studies include all *but*

   a. Moving about on a hard x-ray table
   b. Being rushed through the x-ray procedure
   c. Darkness and noise during fluoroscopy
   d. Enemas or suppositories given before the tests

8. General nursing implications for patients going for any type of radiologic test include all *except*

   a. Helping the patient prepare for waiting by giving him a magazine or other diversion
   b. Making sure that the patient has slippers if he must stand during the test

- **c.** Instructing the patient about any restrictions on food and fluids
- **d.** Listing the complications that may occur

9. General nursing implications when a patient returns from a radiologic test include all *but*

- **a.** Offering a back rub to relieve the discomfort from lying on a hard table
- **b.** Encouraging extra fluids (if pathophysiology allows) when dye was used as a contrast medium
- **c.** Finding out if the patient can eat, and if so, offering some food as soon as possible
- **d.** Keeping the patient on bedrest for four to six hours

10. The specific gravity of urine will be higher than usual after a patient has had all the following x-ray tests *except*

- **a.** K.U.B.
- **b.** Cholangiograms
- **c.** Arteriograms
- **d.** IVP

11. Nursing actions that are routine to help the x-ray technician get a better portable chest x-ray of the patient in bed include all but

- **a.** Helping the patient sit up as straight as possible before the x-ray is done
- **b.** Removing electrodes from the chest before the x-ray
- **c.** Helping the technician place the film holder behind the patient's chest
- **d.** Holding the patient in a fixed position while the x-ray is being done

12. Sally is an adolescent who has a history of severe epigastric pain that is relieved by food or milk. Which of these nursing actions is not routine when Sally has an upper GI series (barium meal)?

- **a.** Keeping Sally on n.p.o. status before the exam
- **b.** Telling Sally that when fluoroscopy is done (as the barium is swallowed) the room will be dark
- **c.** Giving an enema to Sally after the x-rays are completed
- **d.** Informing Sally that the barium sulfate will make the stools light-colored

13. Mr. Somorini is having a barium enema because of slight rectal bleeding. Which of these nursing actions is not routine for the patient having a barium enema?

- **a.** Administration of cathartics or suppositories the evening before the exam
- **b.** Informing Mr. Somorini that he will need to hold the barium in the colon while a series of x-rays are taken
- **c.** Giving a light diet the evening before the x-ray exam
- **d.** Withholding food when Mr. Somorini comes back from x-ray because a second set of pictures are done in three to four hours

14. Mrs. Rigaletti is scheduled for a G.B. series tomorrow morning. Which of the following preparations is not routine the night before a gallbladder series or oral cholecystogram (O.C.G.)?

a. Oral ingestion of six tablets, which contain the contrast medium or dye
b. Low fat diet for evening meal
c. A skin test for sensitivity to iodine
d. NPO after evening meal

15. Mrs. Rigaletti is scheduled to have a cholecystectomy with an exploration of the common bile duct (choledochostomy) because the oral cholecystogram showed gallstones in the common bile duct. When cholangiograms are done during surgery on the biliary tract the dye is usually injected

a. By percutaneous insertion into the common bile duct
b. Directly into the T-tube
c. Intravenously (IVC)
d. Through an endoscope positioned in the gastrointestinal tract

16. Mr. Leonard has just returned to his hospital room after a femoral arteriogram. Which nursing action would be inappropriate?

a. Allowing him to stand if he cannot void in bed
b. Checking vital signs every 15 minutes × 4 times then every 2 hours if vital signs are stable
c. Keeping an ice bag on the puncture site
d. Checking pedal pulses and the color and warmth of the feet when vital signs are done

17. Pain that often requires the use of analgesics is an expected occurence after all these radiologic procedures *except*

a. Mammograms
b. Arthrograms
c. Myelograms
d. Arteriograms

REFERENCES

American Cancer Society. *The Cancer-Related Health Checkup*. New York: American Cancer Society, February 8, 1980.

Arnell, I. & Nassberg, B. ''Administer a Barium Enema Through a Colostomy.'' *Nursing 81*(11):81–83 (February 1981).

Athanasoulis, C. ''Therapeutic Application of Angiograms.'' *New England Journal of Medicine* 302 (20):1117–1125 (May 15, 1980).

Barnett-Wilson, J. "Patients' Responses to Barium X-Ray Studies." *British Medical Journal* 1:6122 (May 13, 1978).

Corbett, J.V. *Laboratory Tests in Nursing Practice*. Norwalk, CT: Appleton-Century-Crofts, 1982.

"Diagnostic Product Information." In *Physician's Desk Reference*, 36th ed. Oradell, NJ: Medical Economics Co. 1982, pp. 3001–3060.

French, R. M. *Guide to Diagnostic Procedures*. New York: McGraw-Hill, 1980.

Gorringe, R. "The Mammography Controversy: A Case for Breast Self-Examination." *Journal of Obstetric Gynecologic and Neonatal Nursing* 7: 7–12 (July/August 1978).

Gray, J. "Radiation Awareness and Exposure Reduction with Audible Monitors." *American Journal of Roentgenology* 133: 1200–1201 (December 1979).

Hales, D. "High Tech in Medicine: Worth the Cost?" *UCSF Magazine* 3:3–14 (March 1980).

Hartfield, M. & Cason, C. "Effects of Information on Emotional Responses During Barium Enema." *Nursing Research* 30:151–155 (May/June 1981).

Health and Human Services. *X-Ray and Vaccination Record*. HHS Publication No. (FDA) 77-8024, 1978.

Johnson, J. & Rice, V. "Sensory and Distress Components of Pain." *Nursing Research* 23:203–209 (May/June 1974).

Kaiser-Permanente Medical Group. *Patient Instruction Sheets for Diagnostic X-Rays*. San Francisco, California, 1981.

McHugh, N., et al. "Preparatory Information: What Helps and Why." *American Journal of Nursing* 82:780–782 (May 1982).

Maphet, Mary. "Radiology: What it Means for Your Patients" *RN* 44:1B–1C (June 1981).

Miller, B. & Keane, C. *Encyclopedia and Dictionary of Medicine, Nursing and Allied Health*, Philadelphia: W. B. Saunders, 1978.

Mongeau, S. & Poirier, H. "X-Rays and Cancer." *World Press Review* 26 (12): 50 (December 1979).

NCRP Report 54. *Medical Radiation Exposure of Pregnant and Potentially Pregnant Women*. Washington, DC: National Council on Radiation Protection and Measurements, 1979.

NCRP Report 48. *Radiation Protection for Medical and Allied Health Personnel*. Washington, DC: National Council on Radiation Protection and Measurements, November 1977.

Ordronneu, N. "Helping Patients in the Radiology Department." *American Journal of Nursing* 80: 1312–1313 (July 1980).

Phipps, W., et al. *Medical-Surgical Nursing Concepts and Clinical Practice*. St. Louis, MO: C. V. Mosby, 1979.

Price, S. & Wilson, L. *Pathophysiology: Clinical Concepts and Disease Processes*. New York: McGraw-Hill, 1978.

Taylor, J. & Ballenger, S. *Neurologic Dysfunction and Nursing Intervention*. New York: McGraw-Hill, 1980.

Tinker, J. "Understanding Chest X-Rays." *American Journal of Nursing* 76: 54–58 (January 1976).

Tucker, S., et al. *Patient Care Standards*, 2nd ed. St. Louis, MO: C. V. Mosby, 1980.

Wilson, P. "Evaluating Chest Films." *Nurse Practitioner* 2: 6–13 (January 1977).

CHAPTER TWO

Tomography and CT Scans

Objectives

1. Contrast and compare the techniques of tomography and computerized axial tomography (CT scan) to routine x-ray images.
2. Indicate the priority nursing intervention when a patient completes a tomogram or CT scan.
3. Compare the usefulness of CT scans to the older diagnostic tests for head and spinal cord abnormalities.
4. Discuss the basic controversy over the use of CT body scans.
5. Compare and contrast preparations needed for infants, children, and adults for CT brain scans.
6. Describe the usual preparations for CT scans of various parts of the body.
7. Describe how PET (positron emission tomography) allows clinicians to examine metabolic functions in a totally new way.

Tomography is a method of body section roentgenography. A specially designed x-ray machine and film holder moves around the patient in an arc, focusing at various angles, each with a slightly different depth. With each change in the angle of the tomography, a selected body plane becomes sharply defined, while the areas above and below the focal point become slightly blurred.

The computerized axial tomographer uses the principle of tomography with the addition of detectors, computers, and a scanner, which make possible a three-dimensional cross-sectional view of the head (CT head scanner) or of other body parts (CT body scanner). Tomograms, also called planigrams or laminagrams, give two-dimensional views.

Cormack, an American physicist, and Hounsfield, an English research engineer, working independently did the research that culminated in the development of the CT scan; they shared a 1979 Nobel Prize for Physiology or Medicine. The Nobel committee acknowledged that no other method of x-ray diagnostics had led to such remarkable success in such a short time.

ADVANTAGES AND DISADVANTAGES

Tomograms and the much more sophisticated CT scans are both noninvasive tests, requiring one skilled technician to operate the machine. Much research is being done to compare the advantages and disadvantages of CT scans with invasive procedures and with sonograms (Chapter 4) and radionuclide scans (Chapter 3) for assessing various pathophysiologic conditions. The major advantage of the CT scan is the exquisite detail of the images.

If a contrast medium is used in conjunction with the tests, as is sometimes done, there are risks associated with the dye injection. (See Chapter 1 on nursing precautions when dye is used.)

A CT scan does have two disadvantages. One is the cost of the test, which must be considered if other less expensive tests can provide satisfactory results. Although CT scans cost approximately $200 to $300 per scan, this may be less than the combined charges of the tests replaced (Haughey, 1981). The second disadvantage of the CT scan is the time of exposure to radiation. Although the amount of radiation is very small, all radiation exposure is cumulative through life. (See Chapter 1 for a detailed discussion on the role of the nurse in relation to the radiation hazards of repeated diagnostic tests.) Yet, when wisely used, the CT scan is a marvel. On the horizon is the use of a scanner that can map not only anatomic structures of the body but also metabolic functions. The newest type of tomography, positron emission tomography (PET), is explained at the end of this chapter.

TOMOGRAMS OF THE LUNGS AND OTHER STRUCTURES

Description and Purposes: As mentioned earlier in this chapter, a tomogram (also called planigram or laminagram) is a special type of x-ray, which takes pictures at various depths of tissue to obtain a cross-sectional view of the body. The procedure takes about 30 minutes, but can be longer for a tomogram of a complete area. Lung tomograms are useful in identifying the exact location of a tumor. (Although ultrasound (Chapter 4) is increasingly being used to identify tumors and fluid in many tissues, it is not effective for tissues with a lot of air, such as the lungs.) Other structures, such as the skeletal system, the sinuses, and various organs, may be effectively viewed by tomographs.

Pretest Nursing Implications

There is no special preparation of the patient. As with any x-ray, all jewelry or other metal must be removed. The procedure does not cause any discomfort, other than that of lying still on the x-ray table. Some patients, however, may be bothered by the noise of the machine.

Posttest Nursing Implications

Patients having tomograms do not require any special aftercare. (See Chapter 1 for ways the nurse can help relieve the anxiety that is often present after diagnostic testing.)

COMPUTERIZED AXIAL TOMOGRAPHY OR EMI SCANNER

Description: CT, CAT scan, Body and Head scans, and EMI scans all refer to the use of computerized axial tomography. The EMI scanner was developed by the *E*lectrical and *M*usical *I*ndustries, a British based group of international companies (Seeram, 1976). Thus, British and Canadian literature are more likely to use the term EMI scanner. American companies are now making scans, too; they use the term CT. CT is usually used, rather than CAT.

Computerized axial tomography uses an x-ray machine that rotates 180 degrees around the patient's head or body. Detectors read the amount of radiation each body tissue or organ absorbs. A computer processes these readings and converts them to a picture shown on a screen, which is stored on discs. The resulting pictures show a three-dimensional cross section of all body parts. The CT scan divides each area of tissue being viewed into an area 3 mm square and 13 mm thick (Miller & Keane, 1978). The results are available in a few minutes. The CT scanner can distinguish almost all types of tissues except nerves. In the older scans of the head, the patient's head was fitted in a rubber bag so there was no cushion or air between the hair and scalp. This is not necessary with the newer scans.

The CT scan, a noninvasive procedure, causes no pain. The patient just lies still while the machine goes around the body. As emphasized before, no risks are entailed, other than being exposed to a small amount of radiation. The procedure takes from 15 to 30 minutes. If a contrast medium is used, the procedure takes 30 to 60 minutes, and there are the usual risks associated with an iodine contrast medium.

Purposes: Around 1972, the first CT scans were used for identifying brain abnormalities and head injuries. The CT was found to be much more valuable in diagnosing problems in the brain than the older x-ray tests (see Chapter 1), such as pneumoencephalograms or cerebral arteriograms. The details available by a CT scan are remarkable. For example, a CT scan can clearly show if a brain abscess is becoming smaller after treatment with antibiotics. CT scans are also used to locate foreign objects in soft tissue, such as the eyes. For example, a piece of metal lodged in an eyeball can be precisely mapped out so the surgeon has to do much less probing. Intracranial lesions, such as neoplasms or hematomas, can be located without a craniotomy. The surgeon thus has a much better understanding of the location and extent of brain pathology before surgery is done.

Body scanners, which were marketed later than head scanners, in 1976, have had a less dramatic and, some would say, a debatable impact. Controversy still remains about how many CT scanners are needed in one community and if each hospital needs a machine. There is also a debate about whether the body scan offers more diagnostic help than other less costly diagnostic tests (van Dyk et al., 1980). This debate has often been carried out in the public press (Saltas, 1979).

Certainly, CT scans of the body are already very useful in research studies. For example, at the University of California at San Francisco, researchers are using the CT body scan to determine the minimum dose of estrogen that will prevent bone degeneration (Hales, 1980). The reader is urged to read current literature to discover the many exciting ways that CT body scans are being used for both diagnostic and research purposes.

Pretest Nursing Implications

Patient Preparation for a Head Scan. Unless a contrast medium is to be used, the patient does not have to maintain n.p.o. status. Some clinicians may even allow clear liquids if a dye is to be used (Bubb, 1981). Wigs and any objects in the hair, such as bobby pins, are removed. The patient can be assured that the procedure is not painful and is much like putting one's head in a hair dryer (Stone, 1977). Note that although the CT is not painful, the thought of having one's head immobilized can be frightening. The person must lie still during the procedure. A two-way intercom allows communication with the x-ray personnel.

Radiopaque dye may be given intravenously to outline the cerebral vessels, if so, the patient may need preparation for this. (See Chapter 1 on how to prepare for potential reactions to dye, which include flushing and possible allergic reaction.)

Preparation of Children. Mills (1980) has developed a booklet to prepare children and their parents for a scan. One suggestion is to encourage the child to play at home by lying still with his head flexed toward his chest. The parent can dim the lights in the room and move an arm around the child's motionless head. By humming softly, the parent gives the child an idea of the sounds he will hear during the test. The child should be taught that he can open and close his eyes but cannot move his head. This preparation may work for children over three. Infants will sleep during the procedure if kept awake and then fed just before the test. The greatest problems will be with toddlers (and confused adults); sedation may be required. Mills (1980) describes, in detail, the procedure for sedation used at the University of Colorado Hospital. Chloral hydrate is usually used, although a mixture of meperidine (Demerol), promethazine (Phenergan), and chlorpromazine (Thorazine) may sometimes be needed. In rare instances, diazepam (Valium) is given intravenously. (See Chapter 8 for a discussion on adverse reactions to sedatives.)

Patient Preparation for CT Body Scans. Scans of the thorax or pelvic regions may or may not require special preparation. The nurse must ask the radiologist what specific preparations are required. A tampon may be used as a vaginal marker. The patient may be required to have a full or empty bladder (van Dyk et al., 1980). A contrast medium may be given to outline various organs. The patient must be assessed for allergies and prepared for a flushing sensation (see Chapter 1). Water is used to inflate the stomach. Also, calcium phosphate tablets may be given for a couple of days before the exam to outline the gastrointestinal tract (Kreel, 1977). The patient may be on a low residue diet for a few days before the exam. Bowel preparations vary in importance with the various parts of the body being scanned. Drugs may be used to decrease peristasis during the test, including propantheline (Buscopan) and glucagon. Synthetic cholecystokin (Sincalide) may also be given to increase peristalsis to cause filling of the GI tract with swallowed Gastrografin (Ruijs, 1979). These medications are given during the procedure and will require an intravenous injection. If a biopsy is planned, guided by the scan, the general nursing implications (discussed in Chapter 6) for invasive procedures, should be heeded.

Posttest Nursing Implications

There are no specific nursing implications related to the scanning procedure. If a radiopaque dye has been given, the nursing implications about dye should be followed. (See the general implications discussed in Chapter 1.) The nurse must be aware of any sedatives or other drugs given as part of the procedure because untoward effects from drugs are always possible. (See the discussion on the side effects of medications used for endoscopic procedures in Chapter 8.) And if invasive measures were done, vital signs and the other assessments described in Chapter 6 would be appropriate.

POSITRON EMISSION TOMOGRAPHY

For positron emission tomography (PET) studies, the patient is injected with a biochemical substance tagged with a radionuclide, which emits positively charged particles. When these radioactive particles combine with the negatively charged electrons normally found in the cells of certain tissue, they emit gamma rays that can be detected by a scanning device. The PET scanner translates the emissions into color-coded images. For example, radioactive glucose can be used to map biochemical activity in the brain (Friedman, 1981). Isotopes used for cardiac studies include oxygen-15, nitrogen-13, and carbon-11 (Ter-Pogossian, 1981). The half-life of the isotopes used is very short so there is very little radiation dosage. Theoretically, any physiologic substance can be tagged and traced as it is metabolized in the body. Much research is being done to make these theoretical possibilities realities.

Emission scanners are sometimes called ECT scans (emission computed tomography) or emission CT scans. They are found only in major medical centers, but the number is rapidly growing both in the United States, Europe, and Japan (Toufexis, 1981). PET is often limited to institutions with access to a cyclotrom for the production of the isotopes; however, some tracers used for emission studies can be shipped prior to use. For example, TC-99m, thallium-201, and gallium-67 are used in PET scans, as well in routine nuclear medicine tests (Kirsch, 1981). See Chapter 3 for more information on conventional radionuclide imaging done routinely in most hospitals.

Questions

1. Tomograms and CT scans are similar in that both tests utilize

a. Fluoroscopic monitors
b. Computers
c. Moving x-ray tubes
d. Three-dimensional pictures as the final product

2. Which of the following is a disadvantage of CT scans as compared to routine x-ray procedures or ultrasound procedures?

a. The number of personnel needed to run the machine
b. The amount of preparation required for the patient
c. The amount of radiation exposure to the patient
d. The lack of detailed images

3. The priority nursing intervention after a patient is finished with a tomogram is to assess

a. Vital signs because of possible adverse effects, such as bleeding
b. Level of anxiety related to potential outcome of procedure
c. Pain level due to the procedure
d. Effects of radiation, such as nausea

4. Baby Jackson has been admitted to an intensive care unit in a large medical center because of head injuries received in an automobile accident. Which of the following tests is considered the most useful for evaluating her head injuries?

a. CT scan
b. Myelogram
c. Pneumoencephalogram
d. Ventriculogram

5. The major controversy surrounding the use of the CT scan as a total body scan is the issue of

a. Radiation hazards
b. Cost compared to benefit
c. Unavailability for most hospitals
d. Pain and discomfort for the patient

6. Preparation for a CT head scan for a three-year-old child is likely to include all the following *except* (no contrast dye is being used)

a. n.p.o. status for three to four hours before the exam
b. Use of sedation 30 minutes before the test
c. Removal of bobby pins or other items in the hair
d. Have the child practice keeping his head still while a humming noise is made

7. Certain types of computerized tomography scanning may require specific patient preparations. Which of the following types of CT scan requires the most physical preparation of the patient?

a. Brain scans **b.** Pelvic scans **c.** Thoracic scans **d.** Abdominal scans

---

REFERENCES

Bubb, D. "Teaching Patients about Ultrasound and CAT Brain Scans." *RN* 44: 64–65 (December 1981).

van Dyk, J. et al. "On the Impact of CT Scanning on Radiotherapy Planning." *Computerized Tomography* 4: 55–65 (April 1980).

Friedman, E. "Imaging Technology Approaches the Frontiers of Physics." *Hospitals* 55: 76–82 (January 1981).

Hales, D. "High Tech in Medicine: Worth the Cost?" *UCSF Magazine* 3: 3–14 (March 1980).

Haughey, C. "What to Say and Do When Your Patient Asks about CT Scans." *Nursing 81* 11: 72–77 (December 1981).

Kirsch, C. M., et al. "Characteristics of a Scanning Multidetector, Single Phonton ECT Body Imager." *Journal of Nuclear Medicine* 22: 726–731 (August 1981).

Kreel, M. D. "Computerized Tomography Using the EMI General Purpose Scanner." *British Journal of Radiology* 50: 2–14 (January 1977).

Miller, B. & Keane, C. *Encyclopedia and Dictionary of Medicine, Nursing and Allied Health.* Philadelphia: W. B. Saunders, 1978.

Mills, G. "Preparing Children and Parents for Cerebral Computerized Tomography." *Maternal Child Nursing* 5: 403–407 (November/December 1980).

Ruijs, S. "A Simple Procedure for Patient Preparation in Abdominal CT." *American Journal of Roentgenology* 133: 551–552 (September 1979).

Saltas, R. "Scanners: Too Many of a Good Thing?" *San Francisco Chronicle and Examiner* 12 (November 4, 1979).

Seeram, E. "The EMI Brain Scanner." *Canadian Nurse* 72: 40–42 (November 1976).

Stone, B. "Computerized Transaxial Brain Scan." *American Journal of Nursing* 77: 1601–1604 (October 1977).

Toufexis, A. "A Brainy Marvel Called PET." *Time* 118:74 (September 14, 1981).

Ter-Pogossian, B. "Positron-Emission Tomography in Cardiac Evaluation." *Hospital Practice* 16: 93–103 (November 1981).

CHAPTER THREE

Diagnostic Tests Using Radionuclides or Radioisotopes

Objectives

1. Differentiate between the use of common radionuclides for diagnostic testing and for therapy.
2. Compare and contrast the procedures used for in vitro and in vivo testing.
3. Explain why pregnant women and children are advised not to have radionuclide studies if other nonradioactive tests can suffice.
4. State the general nursing implications for preparing a patient for any organ scan with technetium (Tc-99m).
5. State the major use of a bone scan done with radionuclides.
6. Explain the purposes of doing a gallium scan in a patient with a fever of undetermined origin.
7. Plan a teaching program for a patient who is to have a radioactive iodine uptake in a couple of weeks.
8. Describe the nursing functions when a patient has a Schilling test.

All of the tests covered in this chapter are done in the nuclear medicine department. The terms radionuclide and radioisotope are both used to describe the radiopharmaceuticals that are used for diagnostic tests at the nuclear medicine department. Often in general practice, the older term radioisotope is still used. However, recent literature uses the more precise term radionuclides, and this term will be used in this chapter. The term radionuclides implies that the element has a nucleus that has been made radioactive.

In diagnostic nuclear medicine, the radionuclide is given to the patient and the radiation emitted from a particular organ is measured. The basic rationale for the use of radionuclides is to observe the function of an organ—not the structure.

RADIONUCLIDES AS RADIOACTIVE ELEMENTS

Radiation occurs where there is a lack of stability in the nuclei of atoms. As the atom spontaneously disintegrates, radiation is emitted in the form of alpha, beta, and gamma rays. Some of the man-made radionuclides are purified so that only gamma rays are emitted. About 50 of the roughly 350 isotopes of all elements in nature are naturally radioactive (Holum, 1979). Isotopes of an element are slightly different molecular forms of the same chemical element. The discovery that certain natural elements were radioactive was made in 1896 by Becquerel, who was working with uranium compounds. In 1903, Becquerel shared a Nobel prize with Marie Curie and Pierre Curie, who discovered another naturally occuring radioactive substance, radium. The unit used to measure the activity of radionuclides is the microcurie named in honor of the Curies.

In the early part of this century, scientists discovered that it was possible to make naturally nonradioactive elements radioactive, by bombarding the nucleus with subatomic fragments to make it unstable. The invention of the cyclotron (atom smasher) in 1931 made it possible to make many elements radioactive. Some of these man-made radionuclides, such as Iodine-131 (I-131), have been used extensively for therapy and diagnostic testing. Therapy with Iodine-131, for cancer of the thyroid, was begun in 1943; a time when both peaceful and war uses of nuclear products were being explored. The use of I-131 for cancer of the thyroid was dubbed the ''atomic cocktail'' (Myers & Wagner, 1974). Because of the length of its half-life, I-131 is infrequently used for diagnostic tests. Newer shorter lived substances have replaced I-131, as discussed later.

USE OF RADIONUCLIDES AS THERAPEUTIC AGENTS

This chapter focuses on the use of radionuclides for diagnostic tests, but it should be pointed out that radionuclides are also used frequently in therapy. The two most commonly used radionuclides are I-131, used to treat some cases of thyroid cancer and hyperthyroidism, and Phosphorous-32 (P-32), used to treat certain malignancies of the bone and bone marrow, such as metastatic bone disease from the prostate or breast and chronic myelogenous and lymphocytic leukemias (Brunner, 1980). Phosphorous-32 is also used to treat polycythenia vera.

METHODS OF DIAGNOSTIC TESTING WITH RADIONUCLIDES

In Vitro Testing

With in vitro testing (sample testing), the radionuclide is given intravenously or orally, and at a later date, samples are taken from the blood and/or urine. Blood volume studies, red blood cell studies, and Schilling test are all examples of tests that use samples, not scans, to measure radionuclides. Sample tests are covered at the end of this chapter, with specific points about nursing implications. Although radioactive iodine uptake (RAI) may also involve the collection of urine samples, it is primarily an in vivo test because the radioactivity of the thyroid gland is measured with a counter. See Table 4 for a list of in vitro testing.

TABLE 4. IN VITRO SAMPLING TESTS

Test	Example of Radionuclide Used	Timing of Test after Dosage	Special Preparation
Red Blood Cells			
Compatibility	Cr-51	1 hour	Blood drawn from patient, then reinjected after tagged
Survival and sequestration	Cr-51	3–4 weeks	Blood samples drawn 2 to 3 times a week
Blood Volume Studies			Blood drawn from patient, then reinjected after tagged
RBC	Cr-51		Record height and weight
Plasma Volume	Radioiodinate serum albumin (RISA)		Must have normal hydration
Schilling Test (test for absorption of B_{12})	B_{12} tagged with Co-57 (oral)		n.p.o. status before test; urine saved for 24 hours; see text for other details, such as administration of B_{12} IM by nurse

In Vivo Testing

The in vivo method (organ scan or scintogram) of measuring the amount of radionuclide in the body is done by organ scanning. See Table 5 for a list of in vivo testing. The scan of an organ is referred to as a scintogram because a scintillation camera is used to make a scan or picture. The scintillation camera, which became available in 1964, has made testing with radionuclides a very useful method of diagnostic testing. The patient is given a radionuclide compound (radiopharmaceutical) intravenously, orally, or by inhalation, depending on the organ to be scanned. Minutes or hours later, or sometimes the following day, the scintillation camera takes a radioactivity reading from the target organ and feeds these readings into a computer. The computer translates these readings into a two-dimensional image or scan. The scintogram is printed in a gray scale so there is more variation than in a black-and-white picture. These varying shades of gray show the relative distribution of the radionuclide in the different parts of the organ. Although the scan is viewed by the human eye, there is little discrepency among observers in interpreting the variations of gray (Chang & Blau, 1979). Very dark spots of the scintogram are called ''hot spots'' because more of the radionuclide was deposited in that spot. Parts of the tissue that do not pick up the radionuclide are seen as light colored areas. Spots without radionuclide uptake are cold spots or cold nodules. Interpretation of the scintogram is done by a physician trained in nuclear medicine, and a verbal report of the scan is put in the patient's chart. Some common findings on scintograms will be discussed for each specific scan covered in this chapter. In general, imaging with radionuclides is most useful where there is disturbance of function rather than a structural defect.

TABLE 5. IN VIVO TESTING (ORGAN SCANS OR SCINTOGRAMS)

Scan	Examples of Radionuclides Type and Route	Timing of Scan after Dosage	Special Preparation
Bone	Tc-99m tagged phosphate compounds (IV)	2–4 hours (takes 1 hour to scan entire body)	Push fluids 2–4 hours before Void before ?Bowel prep
Brain			
Perfusion	Tc-99m pertechnetate (IV)	Immediately	None
Static views	Tc-99m glucoheptenate (IV)	Immediately 15 minutes 1–4 hours	None
	Radio-iodinated human serum albumin (RIHSA) (IV)	18–48 hours	None
Cardiac			
For infarction	Tc-99m pyrophosphate (IV) (Th-201) (IV)	90 minutes to 3 hours	
Perfusion scan	(Th-201) (IV)	3–5 minutes; also in 3–6 hours	
Ejection/fraction studies	Albumin or RBCs tagged with Tc-99m	Immediate with first pass analysis	
Gated-cardiac pool imaging	Same as above	Continuous over 2 hours	
Hepatobiliary			
Liver and spleen (reticuloendothelial cells)	Tc-99m sulfur colloid	10 to 15 minutes	None
Gallbladder	Tc-99m with HIDA or PIPIDA (IV) Tc-99m DISIDA (IV) (Hepatolite)	Immediate and intervals to 24 hours	n.p.o. status for 2 hours before Fat restriction during time of test
Lung			
Perfusion	Tc-99m with albumin (IV)	15 minutes	None
Ventilation	Xe-133 (inhalation) Kr-85 (inhalation)	Immediate Immediate	None None

(*continued*)

TABLE 5. *(Continued)*

Scan	Examples of Radionuclides Type and Route	Timing of Scan after Dosage	Special Preparation
Renal[a]			
Perfusion	Tc-99m DTPA, DSMA Glucoheptanate (IV #1)	Immediate (20 minutes)	Hydrate as ordered
Static views	As above	Up to 4 hours	
Function	I-131 or I-123 tagged to orthoiodohippurate (IV #2)	Immediate and up to 1 hour as continual scan	Hydrate as ordered
Thyroid			
Screening	Tc-99m pertechnetrate (IV)	30 minutes	n.p.o. status 8 hours before and 2 hours posttest
	I-123 (oral)	24 hours	No iodine for 4 weeks pretest
RAI (radioactive iodine uptake)	I-123 or I-131 (oral)	2 hours, 6 hours 24 hours	As above; see text
Total Body Scans			
Inflammatory lesions and neoplasms	Gallium citrate, Ga-67 (IV)	4–6 hours and 24–72 hours or longer	May have bowel prep before
Inflammatory only	Tagged leukocytes with In-111 (IV)	4–24 hours	None

[a]*A triple renal study uses two intravenous injections to obtain perfusion, static views, and excretory function of the kidney.*

See Chapter 2 for a discussion on positron emission tomography (PET), which combines the use of radionuclides with tomography to study in a very sophisticated way both the structure and the function.

Types of Radionuclides Used in Diagnostic Testing

In the past, iodine-131 (I-131) was used not only for diagnosis and therapy for thyroid disorders, but also as a radioactive tag carried to other organs. For example, rose bengal can be tagged with I-131. When the rose bengal is excreted by the liver into the biliary tract, the radioactive substance outlines the hepatobiliary system. Other forms of iodine are also used as radionuclides, including I-123, which has a half-life of 13 hours compared to a half-life of eight days for I-131. (The significance of half-life will be discussed in the section on hazards.) Other radionuclides, such as gallium and thallium, are used for certain types of scanning. Sodium chromate (Cr-51) is used to tag red blood cells, and cobalt (Co-57) is used to tag vitamin B_{12} for the Schilling test. Although various radionuclides are useful for certain tests, technetium (Tc-99m) is the most commonly used for nuclear medicine diagnostic testing (Myers & Wagner, 1974).

Technetium. There are several isotopes of technetium, and all are naturally radioactive. A very unstable form of technetium, Tc-99m, has a half-life of only six hours (Holum, 1979). Technetium-99m is combined with various compounds, which carry the radionuclide to various target organs. For example, bone uses most of the phosphorous in the body, so Tc-99m combined with pyrophosphate is used for a bone scan. Technetium-99m combined with albumin is used as a lung scan because the radio-tagged albumin disperses in the pulmonary precapillary arterioles. Other compounds can carry Tc-99m to other specific organs, such as the hepatobiliary system, thyroid, or brain. If Tc-99m is given without another compound (straight), it is excreted in the urine and in the saliva. Thus, straight Tc-99m can be used to study the parotoid glands or immediate flow through the cerebral vessels. Technetium-99m is always administered intravenously. The timing of the scans after the administration of the radionuclide will depend on the target organ to be viewed. Some organs may take up the substance in a few hours so scans will be done relatively soon while others may not be done for 24 hours or longer.

RADIATION HAZARDS FROM RADIONUCLIDES

The radiation hazard from radionuclide diagnostic testing is very slight because the doses used are usually very small. Also, duration is brief because of the short half-life of the radionuclides used. It was mentioned earlier that the curie (Ci) is the unit used to measure the activity of radionuclides. The curie is based on the radioactivity of a standard gram of radium. The dosages used in therapy are in millicurie levels (1/1000 of a curie). In contrast, dosage levels for the radiopharmaceuticals used for diagnostic testing are in microcurie levels (1/1000 of a millicurie). Thus, the radiation from diagnostic testing is roughly a thousand times less than with therapy (Rummerfield, 1970). When millicurie levels are being used for therapy, other patients and personnel should be protected from the radiation in the patient. The National Council on Radiation Protection and Measurements (1977) has specific guidelines that the hospital *shall* follow when therapy is being done with radionuclides. The guidelines for diagnostic procedures are less complicated than those for therapeutic procedures; however, nuclear medicine personnel must take precautions in handling samples. If urine or fecal matter must be saved for sample testing, the worker should wear water proof gloves when putting the samples in containers or in cleaning bedpans. If urine can be disposed of by diluting it in the sewage system, then no special precautions are needed. Thus, from a nursing point of view, the usual precaution with urine is not to touch the urine, and if samples need to be obtained, water proof gloves should be worn to handle the sample. See the discussion under Posttest Nursing Implications. Exposure to other patients or personnel is not a major problem when radionuclide testing is done. If patients who have had radiopharmaceuticals administered are to remain in the nuclear medicine department, there must be a separate waiting room provided and children should not be allowed as visitors in this room. (NCRP Report 48, 1977). Because the dosage of the substance is very small and half-life short, there is usually no problem in having a patient come back in the unit to wait for later scans.

Waste Disposal for Diagnostic Testing Materials

The minimal radiation hazard from radionuclide diagnostic testing is brief because the half-life of most diagnostic radiopharmaceuticals is very short. Half-life is the time in which it takes a radioactive element to lose half of its radioactivity. An unstable radioactive element continuously disintegrates but some take much longer than others to "physically decay." Iodine-123 has a half-life of only 13 hours, compared to eight days for Iodine-131. Technectium-99m has a half-life of only six hours and disposal is not a problem. In dramatic contrast, radium has a half-life of 1590 years (Holum, 1979). In addition to less exposure for the patient, the shorter the half-life, the less the problem of waste disposal. For nuclear medicine diagnostic testing, the waste disposal problem is not acute because wastes can be held until physical decay occurs.

Radionuclides as Low Level Radioactive Wastes

Because radiation from any source is cumulative, it should always be kept at a minimum for patients, personnel, and the general public. The Nuclear Regulatory Commission grants a license to a physician or an institution to do research, therapy, or diagnostic testing with radioactive material. Specific standards must be maintained, and they are the responsibility of a person designated as the Radiation Protection Officer.

Problems with a Long Half-Life. Large research centers may conduct research that involves the use of Carbon-14, which has a half-life of 5750 years. Radioactive waste that has a very long half-life is picked up by private carriers and taken to three sites for dumping in Nevada, South Carolina, or Washington. (Nuclear plants have their own waste disposal systems.) These three dumping sites may not be enough as more radionuclides are used in testing. For example, when the Washington site was temporarily closed, research centers such as Harvard had to curtail studies that used radioactive materials with long half-lives (*Time Magazine,* 1979). The Nuclear Regulatory Commission is currently working on plans to open up dumping sites in other states for the use of hospitals and other producers of low-level radioactive wastes. The nurse as a health professional, and as a concerned citizen, should keep abreast of what regulations the government provides for all nuclear wastes because the health of entire communities may be threatened when rigid controls are not followed.

Radionuclide Diagnostic Testing during Pregnancy and Childhood

Radiation destroys or alters cells as they go through the dividing stages of growth. In the fetus, and to a lesser degree in the child, cell growth is rapid; thus, many of their cells are vulnerable to alteration by radiation. (This of course is why radiation is used as a therapeutic agent for cancer cells, which are dividing and growing at an increased rate.)

As a general rule, radionuclides are not used for diagnostic testing during pregnancy if other tests can suffice. Although the amount of radioactivity in diagnostic testing is very small it is considered prudent to protect the fetus from any radiation whenever possible. As with x-rays, elective diagnostic tests using radionuclides should be done during menses or within 10 to 14 days after onset of menses for women who could become pregnant (National Council on Radiation Protection and Measurement, 1979). Children should also be protected from radionuclide testing if at all possible. Nursing mothers should not nurse a child during the time of the testing. The risks and benefits for a specific individual are determined by the patient's physician. Eymontt (1977) states that technetium is considered safe for children and for pregnant women. The limits of conservatism may vary in different settings and is sometimes controversial.

Newer Techniques for Radionuclides

A new technique to make radionuclides even safer is a method called fluorescent excitations analysis (FEA), developed at the Lawrence Livermore Radiation Laboratory in conjunction with the University of California at San Francisco (Hales, 1980). This technique uses radionuclides that are "excited" or turned on to emit signals only when the radionuclides reaches the target organ. The radioactivity is only emitted for a short time. With the conventional radionuclide there is a small amount of radiation to the circulatory system as it goes to the target organ and to the bladder as the radionuclide is excreted. Although the radiation from diagnostic radionuclides is very small, it is part of the cumulative amount for the individual. Fluorescent excitations analysis is being researched to make diagnostic radionuclide as safe as possible.

PRETEST NURSING IMPLICATIONS

Relieving Anxiety About the Test

The nurse should be familiar with the particular procedure being used for the test so that the patient's questions can be answered. If the patient is not sure why the test is needed, the nurse can help the patient obtain the correct information from his or her physician. The nurse can assure the patient that the scans do not hurt. The nurse should also inform the patient that he or she will have to lie still during the scan, but the positioning is usually not uncomfortable. The scans may take from 30 to 60 minutes. The machine makes clicking noises at times. Some scanners can be brought to the patient's bedside, but usually it is preferable to do the scan in the nuclear medicine department. Because there is no radiation hazard from the scan, a mother can accompany her child. Some patients may need a sedative or pain medication before the scan, but this is not a common practice. Sedatives do not interfere with the test. Most of the radionuclides are given intravenously so the patient should be told that a venipuncture will be done in the nuclear medicine department. All of the Tc-99m compounds used for organ scans are given intravenously. Iodine compounds may be given orally or intravenously, depending on the test. For some lung studies, the radio-tagged substance is inhaled.

Timing of Scans

The length of time between the administration of the radioisotope and the scan varies, depending on the type of scan (see Table 2). A member of the nuclear medicine department notifies the nurse of the specific time the patient should return for the scan, or if the patient is to remain in the nuclear medicine department for the entire time of the test. Patients should know if they are to stay in the nuclear medicine department for an extended length of time. For outpatients, the patient may be given the radiopharmaceutical and told when to return for the scan.

Reassuring about Radiation Safety

The nurse needs to fully understand the standard procedures for diagnostic radionuclide testing in a specific setting so the patient is not confused about inconsistencies. (See the discussion under posttest care for some variations in the methods of waste disposal.) The nurse can reassure the patient that the dose of radiation used for diagnostic testing is very small and all necessary precautions for safety are being taken. It may also be helpful to point out that only the radioisotope is radioactive. The scintillator acts as a detector of the radiation emitted *from* the patient as opposed to a regular x-ray machine, where radiation is emitted from the machine to penetrate through the body. Thus, the long time, sometimes as much as an hour, spent in front of a scintillator does not cause any radiation effects as would long exposure to an x-ray machine. The clicking sound of the scintillator reflects only measurements of radioactivity already present. (Even health workers may need education about the relative safety of procedures done in the nuclear medicine department.)

Physical Preparation of the Patient before a Scintogram

Usually no physical preparation is necessary before the scan. With almost all scans, the patient can eat and take any needed medications. Enemas may be needed for certain scans. (See the discussion about each test and Table 4 for specific details.) Of course, any jewelry or metal should be removed from the area to be scanned.

POSTTEST NURSING IMPLICATIONS

Assessing for Adverse Reactions

Major assessments are not needed after most scanning procedures. If a stress test was done as part of a thallium scan for coronary perfusion, there are specific posttest considerations (see Chapter 7 on stress tests). If the radionuclide was given intravenously, and almost all are, the site of the needle puncture should be assessed for inflammation. Warm packs can be used for any phlebitis that develops. The medications used for testing are unlikely to cause any side effects.

Relieving Posttest Anxiety

As discussed in Chapter 1, the nurse is often able to act as a ''sounding board'' for the patient who has anxiety about his condition. The results of the scan are not usually available for a day or two, so the nurse can help the patient formulate specific questions to ask the physician. For example, if a liver scan was done to assess for possible metastasis, the person will be very anxious while awaiting the results. The nurse can help the person ventilate feelings and identify the major areas of concern regarding choices about treatments, etc.

Encouraging Fluids

As noted in the pretest preparations, most of the scans do not require any restrictions in diet, either before or after the scan. If there are no contraindications, the patient should be encouraged to drink extra fluids to help expedite radionuclide excretion.

Disposing of Urine

Although the amount of diagnostic radionuclide excreted in the urine is very low, urine should not be used for any laboratory tests. Patients should be told to flush the toilet three times after voiding. Rubber gloves are recommended if the urine must be handled (National Council on Radiation Protection and Measurement, 1977). The nuclear medicine department must supply the information about the timing of the precautions with urine, based on the half-life of the radionuclide used.

Some hospitals have developed specific guidelines and appointed safety advisors for personnel who care for patients confined to bed and who are undergoing nuclear medicine diagnostic procedures. Infants also pose a problem for disposal of wastes because the nurse must handle the urine. At San Francisco General Hospital (1980) the following guidelines have been instituted:

1. Wear disposable gloves (not sterile ones) when handling wastes.
2. Flush the toilet three times after excreta is discarded.
3. Rinse reusable containers twice before doing general cleaning.
4. Rinse disposable containers twice before discarding in the general waste.
5. Wash hands with gloves on. Remove gloves and wash hands again. Dispose of gloves in general waste.
6. For infants and incontinent patients use disposable diapers, wear disposable gloves when changing diapers, and discard gloves and waste as above.

The reader is encouraged to talk to nuclear medicine personnel in a specific setting to obtain accurate up-to-date information about guidelines used for patients undergoing tests with radionuclides. The nurse should not unduly alarm patients. If some urine is accidentally spilled or touched, this is not an emergency. Immediate disposal of the waste is not of the same urgency as when patients have therapy with radioactive substances. The nurse should act in a prudent manner so that any and all exposure to radiation is minimized. (See Chapter 1 for more discussion on the radiation hazards for health workers.)

SPECIFIC TYPES OF SCANS

BONE SCANS

Description: For a bone scan, Tc-99m pyrophosphate is given intravenously. In two to four hours, the radionuclide will concentrate in the bone tissue. It takes about an hour for the scintillation camera to scan the entire body, front and back. If there is increased bone activity, the bone tissue will take up more of the radionuclide. The scan will outline areas of osteoblastic and osteolytic processes in the bones, such as malignant tumors or osteoporosis.

Purposes: A bone scan is most often done to check for silent metastasis to the bone. A metastatic lesion in the bone will show up on a scan about six months earlier than on a regular x-ray (Robinson, 1979). Bone scans may be done on a routine basis after detection of malignancies of the breast or prostate because bone metastasis is a strong possibility with these malignancies (Price & Wilson, 1978).

Pretest Nursing Implications

The patient must void before a bone scan so the pelvic bones can be seen. Also, the patient may need an enema or laxative. Fluids should be pushed for two to four hours before the test to ensure that the patient is well hydrated.

BRAIN SCANS

Brain scans are done as perfusion scans and static views of the brain tissues. A cerebral perfusion scan is done 30 seconds after the intravenous injection of Tc-99m. If straight Tc-99m is used, some of it will be excreted in the saliva; the patient must not touch the saliva and then put his or her hands near his or her head. Technetium-99m pertechnetate static scans of the brain are done at intervals, such as 15 minutes, 1 hour, and 24 hours. If a lesion has damaged the blood brain barrier, the radionuclide will localize in that area. The blood brain barrier is a complex system of membranes and fluid spaces, which keep substances in the blood from diffusing into the brain tissue. Tumors and other lesions destroy this protective barrier; consequently, more of the radionuclide diffuses into the brain tissue. Radio-iodinated human serum albumin (RIHSA) may also be used to evaluate changes in the blood brain barrier.

GALLIUM SCANS

Gallium citrate (Ga-67) is useful in diagnostic scanning because gallium localizes in inflammatory lesions and in certain neoplastic tumors. The exact mechanisms of gallium accumulation in neoplastic and inflammatory lesions have not yet been established (Pelosi et al., 1980). A gallium scan may be used to detect a hidden abscess or metastatic nodules. Ultrasound (Chapter 4) may show the presence of a pelvic mass, but is not useful in determining if a mass is benign or malignant. A gallium scan can be a complementary procedure in studying the nature of a mass found by other diagnostic means. Gallium scans may be done two to three days after the administration of the Ga-67 to assess neoplasms. For inflammatory lesions, the initial scan is done in four to six hours.

Pretest Nursing Implications

Enemas or laxatives are sometimes given before a gallium scan to empty the gastrointestinal tract. The intestinal tract collects gallium and confusing results may occur if there are shadows in the gastrointestinal tract. Not all institutions require bowel preps.

INDIUM SCANS

Indium (In-111) is used to label leukocytes, which then go to infected areas of the body. In contrast to gallium, In-111–labeled leukocytes are taken up by neither neoplastic lesions nor by noninfected wounds that are healing (Thakur, 1981). Any infected area in the body can be visualized in 4 to 24 hours. Indium is also used to label platelets and red blood cells for other types of studies. There is no special preparation of the patient.

GALLBLADDER SCANS

Description: The older technique to screen the biliary tract used rose bengal or BSP dye tagged with I-131. These substances are excreted by the liver into the biliary tree and concentrate in the gallbladder. The newer and very promising method of evaluating biliary function is with Tc-99m combined with chemicals, such as HIDA and PIPDA (Eikman, 1979). These newer scans are done immediately and at intervals over a 24-hour period. *Purposes*: When information about organs adjacent to the gallbladder is not desirable, the radionuclide scan of the hepatobiliary tree may become the first procedure done to evaluate acute cholecystitis (Whalen, 1979). Hepatobiliary scans are also done in conjunction with ultrasound and x-ray studies of the gallbladder for chronic cholecystitis or for assessment of obstructive jaundice.

Pretest Nursing Implications

The patient is kept on n.p.o. status for a few hours before the test. The patient may eat after the initial sonogram but fats arc restricted during the 24-hour test period to decrease rapid emptying of the gallbladder.

LIVER SCANS

Hepatobiliary scans are used primarily to note biliary function; however, liver function is assessed, too, because the agents used to outline the biliary tree are excreted by the liver. Many different radiopharmaceuticals can be used for specific liver scans to assess the reticuloendothelial system or the structural changes in cirrhosis. A liver scan is a common procedure for patients where liver metastasis is suspected. Technetium-99m is combined with a sulfur colloid to assess for neoplasms in the liver (Snow et al., 1979). The scan is done 10 to 15 minutes after the radionuclide is injected intravenously. No special preparation is needed.

LUNG SCANS

Lung scans may be done either as perfusion studies or as ventilation scans. Perfusion studies use albumin tagged with Tc-99m, which disperses in the pulmonary precapillary arterioles. Perfusion lung scans are used to evaluate the possibility of pulmonary embolisms (Price & Wilson, 1978). Ventilation lung scans are done with radioactive gas. The patient inhales a bolus of Xenon-123. The lungs are then scanned for about five minutes to determine how much gas enters each lobe of the lung and how long it takes the gas to be expelled. Krypton is another radioactive gas used for ventilation studies (Robinson, 1979). Radionuclide perfusion studies and ventilation studies are usually correlated with other pulmonary function tests (see Chapter 5) and blood gas studies. The lung scan is inappropriate when searching for a tumor, which is almost always more evident on a chest film—unless the tumor has invaded pulmonary vessels (Silberstein, 1980). There is no special preparation of the patient.

CARDIAC SCANS

Infarction Scans. A new test for detecting myocardial infarction uses Tc-99m pyrophosphate (the same compound used in bone scans). Thallium (Th-201) may also be used for infarction scans. If there is an infarction in the myocardium, there will be an increased uptake of the radionuclide in this "hot" spot. The scan of the myocardium is done one-and-a-half to three hours after the intravenous injection of the radionuclide. The test can be done at the patient's bedside to prevent exertion on the part of the patient. This test is reported to be more than 90 percent accurate in diagnosing transmural infarctions. For diagnosing subendocardial infarctions the test is 60 to 70 percent accurate (Disch, 1980). The hot spot myocardial imaging test is most helpful one to three days after the infarction. This test may become useful in cases where the more traditional ways of diagnosing myocardial infarction, cardiac enzymes and ECG readings (Chapter 5), have not given enough information.

Perfusion Scans. A thallium scan is also useful for evaluating coronary perfusion. A thallium scan may show the site of an old infarction or demonstrate partial obstructions to coronary blood flow. Poorly perfused regions of the myocardium will show up as low levels of thallium uptake (Disch, 1980). A stress test may be done as part of a thallium scan because coronary perfusion may only decrease with a certain amount of exertion. Research has suggested that combining a thallium scintogram with a stress test improves the prognostic ability of the tests, particularly in patients who have multivessel disease (Smeets et al., 1981). If a stress test is done in conjunction with the thallium scan, nursing care after the test will include careful assessment of the cardiac status of the patient. (See Chapter 7 for a complete description of stress testing.)

Other Types of Cardiac Imaging. Sophisticated studies of heart function, including wall motion studies and ejection fraction studies, can be done by tagging red blood cells or albumin with Tc-99m. For ejection fraction studies, the scanning is done as the radionuclide passes through the heart. The amount of radionuclide ejected with each heart beat can be calculated, and any shunting can be detected. The function of the valves can also be assessed with the first "pass through" of the radionuclide. Scans done continuously over one or two hours are done in conjunction with electrographic monitoring of cardiac function. Signals from the ECG trigger the scintillation camera to record the flow of blood at precise times in the cardiac cycle. The procedure is called gated-cardiac imaging because the series of images of blood flow through the heart can be studied in sequence. At precise times in the cardiac cycle the scintillator is turned on to record function.

These gated types of images are used to assess ventricular function. For example, a postinfarction patient can be evaluated to determine if developing congestive failure is due to overall poor contractibility or to a regional abnormality, such as a ventricular aneurysm (Wenger et al., 1980).

Another use of radionuclides for cardiac scanning is to screen asymptomatic children with murmurs of questionable significance. Cardiac scanning by nuclear imaging may help avoid the need for angiocardiography (Robinson, 1979). (See Chapter 7 for a discussion on cardiac catheterization, which may be a follow-up after nuclear scanning.) Note also that isotopes are used in conjunction with PET (positron emission tomography) scans to do cardiac evaluations. (See Chapter 2 for a discussion on PET.)

Pretest Nursing Implications

If a stress test is to be done with a thallium scan, there are very specific preparations for the stress test component (see Chapter 7 for stress tests). For other cardiac scans, there is no special preparation, except for the general nursing implications discussed in the beginning of this chapter. Nuclear cardiac studies may be done in specialized care units, such as coronary care settings, as well as outpatient settings.

RENAL SCANS

Scans of the kidneys evaluate both renal perfusion and function. Technetium-99m is tagged to a compound such as DTPA. The tagged compound is administered intravenously, and a series of scans are taken to assess the dynamic perfusion of the kidneys. Static scans are taken from 20 minutes up to four hours to assess the structure of the kidneys. Another type of compound orthoiodohippurate (Hippuran) tagged with radioactive iodine can be given as a second intravenous injection so continuous images can be obtained over approximately an hour to measure the time it takes to travel through the cortex and pelvis of each kidney. The times of uptake, transient, and excretion of the radionuclide by each kidney can be plotted on a graph called an isotope renogram curve. Plotted curves are compared to normal reference curves to determine abnormalities in either kidney. The use of two intravenous injections to obtain the perfusion, structure, and excretory ability of the kidneys is sometimes called a triple renal study.

Intravenous pyelogram (IVP) involves the use of a radiopaque dye to evaluate the excretory ability of the renal system (see Chapter 1 for IVP). For patients allergic to the contrast medium used for IVP, renograms can be used as a substitute to assess the excretory pattern. The use of renal imaging to assess renal dysfunction is used in conjunction with various other diagnostic studies. Renal biopsies (Chapter 6) are sometimes done in conjunction with renal scans.

Pretest Nursing Implications

See the general implications in the introduction. In addition, the patient should be well hydrated. For aftercare, see the discussion on safety precautions for disposing of urine.

THYROID SCANS

Several different isotopes of iodine are used for thyroid scans. Iodine, such as I-123, can be given either orally or intravenously. Scans of the thyroid are done to assess nodules, which may be felt in the thyroid gland. Benign nodules appear as "warm" spots on the scan because they tend to take up the radionuclide. Conversely, malignant tumors appear as "cold" spots because they do not tend to take up the radionuclide. The actual presence of a malignancy must still be determined by a biopsy. (A special type of scanning of the thyroid called a radioactive iodine uptake (RAI) is discussed in a separate section because the RAI is different from organ scans in general.)

When screening someone with no symptoms of thyroid problems, thyroid scans can be done with Tc-99m because the screening can be done faster with less radiation exposure due to the short half-life of Tc-99m. Thyroid scans are also done on people who have no thyroid problems, but do have a history of x-ray radiation to the face and neck. Until the late 1950s, x-ray therapy was used in the treatment of acne and thymus gland disorders, and this past radiation may promote malignant growths in the thyroid gland (Guimond & Wilson, 1979).

See the next section on RAI for the restrictions on iodine uptake before thyroid scans with radioactive iodine.

RAI UPTAKE

For an RAI uptake, the patient is given radioactive iodine either in an oral capsule or intravenously. The uptake by the thyroid gland is measured by a scanner at several time intervals, such as one hour, six hours, and in 24 and 48 hours. A person with hyperthyroidism will have an increased uptake of iodine, perhaps as high as 90 percent. Conversely, the person with hypothyroidism will have a decreased uptake of iodine by the thyroid gland. The values of the RAI uptake are expressed in percentages: the amount of thyroid uptake divided by the amount of the dose given. The reference values vary depending on the locality because normal iodine consumption varies in different locales (Brunner & Suddarth, 1980).

Reference Values:

- Scan (uptake): 1–13% after 2 hours
  2–25% after 6 hours
  15–45% after 24 hours
- Urine with I-123: 37–75% excreted (Med-Physics, 1975)

Pretest Nursing Implications

Because the amount of iodine consumption before the test affects the uptake of radioactive iodine, it is important that the patient not have additional iodine uptake for several weeks before the test. A list of medications currently being taken by the patient should be put on the laboratory request.

As mentioned in Chapter 1, many contrast mediums used for x-ray studies have an iodine base. A patient should have an RAI before studies that use iodine dye. Patients need to be instructed to avoid all sources of iodine. Certain foods, such as kelp and enriched breakfast cereals, are high in iodine. Vitamin preparations may contain iodine, as do most cough syrups. Even suntan lotion and nail polish can be sources of exogenous iodine. Such a small amount of iodine is used for the RAI that it does not cause any allergic problems, even in people who are allergic to iodine. (In contrast, x-ray dyes that contain iodine can cause anaphylactic shock in allergic individuals.)

Posttest Nursing Implications

For some RAI tests, urine samples may be saved for monitoring, but saving urine is not common. If saved, the urine does not need a preservative. The amount of iodine excreted in the urine will depend both on the thyroid uptake and the normalcy of renal function. Adequate fluids should be encouraged for the patient. If urine is to be handled, the precautions discussed earlier should be noted (e.g., wearing rubber gloves).

OTHER ORGAN SCANS

The pancreas, adrenals, and lacrimal ducts are some of the other structures which can be scanned when the appropriate carrying compound is tagged with a radionuclide. Imaging of some glands, such as the pancreas or parathyroid, has been difficult to achieve (Valk et al., 1976). A compound must be specific for the target area. For example, tagged fibrinogen will go to a venous clot and may help assess the presence of a thrombus. Radioactive cholesterol is used to get images of the adrenal gland. The scan of the adrenals is done in two to four days or seven to ten days, depending on the radionuclide used to tag the cholesterol (Robinson, 1979). The reader must consult current literature to obtain data on the newest techniques developed for organ scanning—a dynamic and growing field.

IN VITRO SAMPLING: COMPATABILITY AND RBC SURVIVAL

Sodium chromate (Cr-51) readily binds with the protein of hemoglobin so red blood cells can be tagged to evaluate the rate of hemolysis or red blood cell survival in certain types of hemolytic diseases. A sample of blood is withdrawn from the patient, tagged with the radioactive Cr-51, and injected back into the patient. A collection of blood samples are drawn at various time intervals. One sample may be drawn within one hour to measure comparability and then two to three times a week to assess survival. No special preparation of the patient is required.

BLOOD VOLUME STUDIES

Sodium chromate (Cr-51) is also used to determine blood volume. It is used to tag the RBCs, and radioiodinate serum albumin (RISA) is used to tag plasma. A measured amount of blood is withdrawn from the patient, tagged with radionuclides, and injected back into the patient. After 15 to 30 minutes, samples of blood are drawn and the amount of dilution of the original sample is calculated. The total blood volume of a patient can thus be estimated. It is very important that the hydration of the patient be normal before the blood studies are done. Intravenous solutions will invalidate the test, as will a n.p.o. state. The nurse must record the height and weight of the patient before the test is done.

SCHILLING TEST

The Schilling test is used to assess the ability of the small intestine to absorb vitamin B_{12}. An oral preparation of vitamin B_{12} is tagged with Cobalt-57. The test measures how much of the tagged B_{12} is eliminated in the urine. The patient is given a loading dose of untagged vitamin B_{12} intramuscularly to saturate the cells with B_{12}. The nurse may give this injection several hours before the test. The patient must fast for six to eight hours before the test and for two additional hours after the B_{12} is given. The oral cobalt-tagged vitamin B_{12} is given by the nuclear medicine department personnel. All urine is collected for 24 hours and should be kept on ice. No preservative is needed. If renal function is questionable, the test may last longer. The precautions for urine handling should be noted, as discussed earlier in this chapter.

Reference Values

Eight to 40 percent of the dose of tagged B_{12} should be eliminated in the urine.

Clinical Significance

If urine excretion of the tagged B_{12} is subnormal, the test is repeated with an extract of intrinsic factor given with the oral B_{12}. Intrinsic factor is found in the gastric mucosa and is essential for the proper absorption of vitamin B_{12}. If urine values increase when intrinsic factor is given with B_{12}, a diagnosis of pernicious anemia is made. Other reasons for decreased oral vitamin B_{12} absorption may be due to lack of pancreatic enzymes or an overgrowth of bacteria in the gut so these factors may need to be investigated, too. Some unusual and unexplained anemias may be assessed by bone marrow biopsies. If bone marrow studies are ordered, these are done before any injections of vitamin B_{12} because vitamins change the picture of the bone marrow (see Chapter 6 on bone marrow studies).

Questions

1. Scientists can make a nonradioactive element radioactive (e.g., iodine to I-131 or I-123) by

- **a.** Exposing the iodine to x-rays for a certain period of time
- **b.** Injecting subatomic particles into the nucleus of the iodine atom
- **c.** Mixing the iodine with naturally occuring radioactive substances, such as technetium (Tc-99m)
- **d.** Using a cyclotron to make the nucleus stable

2. Technetium (Tc-99m) is useful as an agent for diagnostic testing because this radioactive element

- **a.** Has a half-life of only two days
- **b.** Can be tagged to go to the brain, bone, liver, or lung

c. Is radioactive only when it reaches the target organ
d. Is excreted only in the urine

3. Scintography involves taking the reading of radioactivity from a body organ and transforming the readings into

a. Audible sounds (Geiger counter)
b. Quantitative measurements
c. A two-dimensional image of the organ
d. A vertical graph

4. The radiation hazard from radionuclide diagnostic testing is much less than when radionuclides are used for therapy because the dose used for diagnostic testing is about

a. Half as much as used in therapy
b. 10 times less than therapy
c. 100 times less than therapy
d. 1000 times less than therapy

5. Which of the following would be a reason to postpone radionuclide diagnostic studies? The woman who is

a. Seven days past onset of menstrual period
b. Breast feeding
c. Menstruating
d. Allergic to iodine

6. Which of the following nursing actions is appropriate in preparing a patient for any organ scan with technetium (Tc-99m)?

a. Explain to the patient that all urine must be monitored after the test
b. Keep the patient on n.p.o. status
c. Explain that the test involves intravenous administration of a very small dose of a radioactive substance
d. Shave the area that will be viewed by the scan

7. The major use of a bone scan done with radionuclides is to detect

a. Silent metastasis from the breast or prostate gland
b. Silent metastasis from the liver or kidney
c. Utilization of phosphorous by the body
d. Fractures

8. Mrs. Lourdes is going to have a gallium scan done this morning because of a fever of undetermined origin (FUO). Gallium is useful as a radionuclide for scintography because gallium localizes in

a. Inflammed tissue or certain types of tumors
b. The lungs
c. The brain and spinal column
d. The hepato-biliary system

9. Mrs. Hunter is scheduled for a radioactive iodine uptake (RAI) in four weeks so she is to have no iodine intake. Which of the following is *not* a potential source of iodine?

a. Suntan lotions
b. Vitamin preparations
c. Contrast medium for x-ray tests
d. Soft drinks, such as colas

10. Mr. Langerdorf is having a Schilling test done today. Which of the following is *not* an appropriate nursing function in regard to this test?

a. Saving all urine for 24 hours after the oral cobalt-tagged B_{12} is given
b. Giving the ordered intramuscular injection of B_{12} as a loading dose before the oral cobalt-tagged B_{12} is given
c. Keeping the patient isolated from other patients because radioactive cobalt is used
d. Using rubber gloves when collecting urine samples.

REFERENCES

Brunner, L. & Suddarth, D. *Textbook of Medical-Surgical Nursing,* Philadelphia: J. B. Lippincott, 1980.

Chang, W. & Blau, M. "Optimization of the Gray Scale for Photo Scanners." *Journal of Nuclear Medicine* 20: 57–59 (January 1979).

Diagnostic Services Utilization Committee, *Guidelines for Diagnostic Tests.* San Francisco: Kaiser Permanente Medical Center, June 1980.

Disch, J. *Diagnostic Procedures for Cardiovascular Disease.* Norwalk, CT: Appleton-Century-Crofts, 1980.

"Dump Slump: It Hurts Nuclear Medicine," *Time Magazine* 114: 102 (October 29, 1979).

Eikman, E. "Radionuclide Hepatobiliary Procedures: When Can HIDA Help?" *Journal of Nuclear Medicine* 20(4): 358–360 (April 1979).

Eymontt, M. & Eymontt, D. "Preparing Your Patient for Nuclear Medicine." *Nursing 77*(7): 46–49 (December 1977).

Guimond, J. & Wilson, S. "Postirridation Thyroid Disorders." *American Journal of Nursing* 79: 1256–1258 (July 1979).

Hales, D. "Imaging—Beyond CT." *UCSF Magazine* 3: 9–10 (March 1980).

Holum, J. *Elements of General and Biological Chemistry,* 5th ed. New York: John Wiley and Sons, 1979.

Medi-Physics, Inc. "Sodium Iolide I-123—Capsules and Solution for Oral Administration-Diagnostic." Package insert by manufacturer. Emeryville, CA, December 1975.

Myers, W. & Wagner, H. "Nuclear Medicine: How It Began." *Hospital Practice* 9(2): 103–113 (March 1974).

NCRP Report 54. *Medical Radiation Exposure of Pregnant and Potentially Pregnant Women.* Washington, DC: National Council on Radiation Protection and Measurements, September 15, 1979.

NCRP Report 48. "Radioactive Nuclides." In *Radiation Protection for Medical and Allied Health Personnel.* Washington, DC: National Council on Radiation Protection and Measurements, November 1, 1977.

Pelosi, M., et al. "Combined Use of Ultrasonography and Gallium Scanning in the Diagnosis of Pelvic Pathology." *Surgery, Gynecology and Obstetrics* 150: 331–336 (March 1980).

Price, S. & Wilson, L. *Pathophysiology: Clinical Concepts of Disease Processes.* New York: McGraw-Hill, 1978.

Robinson, P. J. "Clinical Uses of Isotope Imaging." In *Medical Imaging* (L. Kreel, ed.) Chicago: Year Book Medical Publishers, Inc., 1979.

Rummerfield, P. & Rummerfield, M. "What You Should Know about Radiation Hazards." *American Journal of Nursing* 70: 780–786 (April 1970).

San Francisco General Hospital. *Safety Advisory for Nurses Handling Excreta from Patients Confined to Bed and Undergoing Nuclear Medicine Diagnostic Procedures*. San Francisco, November 1980.

Silberstein, E. "Nuclear Medicine and the Lung: Perfusion and Ventilation." *Basics of Respiratory Disease* 9:5–6 (September 1980).

Smeets, J. P., et al. "Prognostic Value of Thallium-201-Stress Myocardial Scintography with Exercise ECG After Myocardial Infarction." *Cardiology* 68 (Supplement 2): 67–70 (1981).

Snow, J., et al. "Comparison of Scintography, Sonography and Computed Tomography in the Evaluation of Hepatic Neoplasms." *American Journal of Roentgenology* 132: 915–917 (June 1979).

Thakur, M. "New Radionuclides in the Diagnosis of Obscure Infections." *Connecticut Medicine* 45: 302–304 (May 1981).

Valk, P. et al. "Technetium Radiopharmaceuticals as Diagnostic Organ Imaging Agents." *Journal of Chemical Education* 53: 542–543 (September 1976).

Whalen, J. "Newer Imagery Methods of the Abdomen." *American Journal of Roentgenology* 133: 587–615 (October 1979).

Wenger, N. et al. *Cardiology for Nurses*. New York: McGraw Hill, 1980.

CHAPTER FOUR

Diagnostic Ultrasonography

Objectives

1. Explain the differences between A mode, B scans, and ''real-time'' scans as methods of pulse-echo recordings of ultrasound.
2. Describe three clinical situations where the nurse uses the Doppler method of ultrasound for assessment.
3. Describe the necessary preparation of the patient for pelvic and abdominal sonograms.
4. Explain the specific use of echocardiograms as diagnostic tests for cardiac problems.
5. Describe the responsibilities of the nurse when a young child has an echoencephalogram.
6. Explain why ultrasound exams of the thorax are of limited usefulness.

Ultrasound is an exciting new noninvasive risk-free method of diagnostic testing, which uses sound waves to detect physical changes in the patient. Sound is a physical force, and thus is in no way related to x-rays (discussed in Chapter 1), computer axial tomography scans, (discussed in Chapter 2), and the radionuclide scans (discussed in Chapter 3).

Ultrasound, first used in industry to detect flaws in metal, is used as a sonar system to locate objects in the water and for depth sounding of the ocean floor. In addition, it has become a very common diagnostic tool in pregnancy. Ultrasound has also become well-established as a cardiac diagnostic test (echocardiogram) for certain cardiac problems. A newer and very rapidly growing use of ultrasound is to assess various pathologic conditions of the abdomen. Common tests using both the pulse-echo recordings and Doppler methods are covered in this chapter (see Table 6). The Doppler method of assessment is often used by the nurse in obstetric settings and in medical-surgical units.

TABLE 6. ULTRASOUND METHODS USED FOR ASSESSMENT

Method	Examples of Use
A. Pulse-echo methods	
1. A mode (amplitude modulation)	echocardiogram
2. B mode (brightness modulation)	sonograms of fetus, pelvic and abdominal structures
B. Doppler method	
1. Doppler stethoscope	monitoring of fetal heart rate
2. Doppler instrument	monitoring of peripheral pulses

ULTRASOUND AS THERAPY

Although this chapter focuses on the use of ultrasound as a diagnostic tool, ultrasound waves are also used as therapy. Ultrasound, in large and continuous doses, can generate heat in tissues; therefore, ultrasound treatments are used for various kinds of low back pain. Ultrasound has also been tried as a method to promote tissue regeneration. A very new use of ultrasound therapy is treatment of tumors. Research is being started on the use of ultrasound and microwave to generate heat to kill malignant growths (Research Round-up, 1980).

DESCRIPTION

Ultrasonics is part of the science of acoustics that deals with sound waves that are beyond the range of audible sound. The human ear can hear sounds that are of a frequency between 16,000 and 20,000 cycles per second. The unit of frequency is a Hertz (Hz), which is equal to one cycle per second. Thus, ultrasound waves are of a frequency higher than 20,000 Hz (Wells, 1979). Sonograms are done with transducers, which produce sound waves of varying strength or intensity. Intensity is the measure of the strength of a sound wave and is measured as the amount of power per a cross-sectional area. However, more useful to the nurse than figures of frequencies and intensities is the comparison of dosages used in tests. Intensities employed for therapeutic treatment are at least 20 times the intensities used in diagnostic testing (Ziskin, 1980).

For diagnostic purposes, ultrasound waves are sent into the body by a small transducer,[1] pressed against the skin. A transducer changes one form of energy into another. An electric signal from the machine is converted to ultrasound waves. Air almost completely impedes the transmission of the ultrasound waves into the body; thus the transducer must be in good contact with the skin as it is being moved. A lubricant, such as

[1]Technically, the transducer is just the piezo-electric crystal, which does the changing of electric energy to sound waves and vice versa. However, the unit which houses the crystal is also called the transducer in general terms.

mineral oil, glycerin, or a water-based jelly, is used to ensure good contact with the skin. The lubricant is called the coupling agent. When it is difficult to evenly move the transducer over an area (e.g., ultrasound of the neck, scrotum, or breast), the transducer can be supported in a plastic bag of water (Pachaczevsk, 1979). The transducer not only sends the sound waves into the body, it also receives any returning sound waves, which are deflected back as they bounce off various structures. Some sound waves pass through the body. The transducer converts the returning sound waves into electric signals that can then be transformed by a computer in either scans or graphs (pulse-echo methods) or into audible sounds (Doppler method). Regarding sound waves that go through the body, research is just now beginning to look at the "through transmission" technique.

PULSE-ECHO METHOD OF DISPLAYING ULTRASOUND

All of the pulse-echo techniques measure the time it takes the sound waves to reach various structures and return to the transducer. There are various ways that the read out can be done. In the A mode (amplitude modulation) the echoes are displayed in a graphic form, for example, the graph done for an echocardiogram. In the B mode (brightness modulation) the echoes appear as different intensities of brightness. B scans use these dots of brightness to show a two-dimensional cross-sectional view of the various structures. Thus, with a B scan, one can actually see a "picture" of the fetus in the womb, for example. The B scans may be still (static scans) or motion may be added.

REAL-TIME IMAGING

The term "real time" or "real-time imaging" is computer jargon for scanners that are capable of very rapid scanning so that motion can be displayed (Meire, 1977). A still picture with a B scan takes 20 seconds. For upper abdominal sonograms, the patient must lie very still and hold his or her breath so the usual movement of the diaphragm will not interfere with the picture. A scan that has real-time imaging is capable of thirty frames per second. In other words, the real-time scanning is like a movie. A fetus can be seen moving around, sucking a thumb, or other motions. The use of the scanner with rapid sequencing is very valuable in observing heart action. For real-time imaging there is no need for the patient to suspend respiration during the scan. Thus, real-time scanning is better suited for infants, children, or confused adults (James, 1980).

GRAY SCALE

The first sonograms were black and white. In 1979 the gray scale became available. The various shades of gray allow some distinctions among structures, but it is still not precise for each type of tissue. Kreel & Steiner (1979) predict that in a few years computer analysis will be able to specifically identify different tissues to make a very sophisticated scan.

DOPPLER TECHNIQUES

With the Doppler method, returning sound waves are transformed into audible sounds, which can be heard with earphones. Not only are sound waves produced by moving objects, but sound waves bounced off of different moving objects have slightly different frequencies. This technique is used to assess the movement of the opening and closing of the heart valves and the flow of blood. This technique is used for bedside assessments, as well as a laboratory diagnostic aid. The Doppler stethoscope can detect the presence of fetal heartbeats, even when the heartbeat is inaudible by the conventional stethoscope. The Doppler technique can be used as a type of fetal monitoring during labor and delivery. The Doppler technique is also used to monitor the fetus during the OCT (ocytocin challenge test) or the NST (nonstress test), which may be done during the last trimester of pregnancy. (See Chapter 9 for tests in pregnancy.)

In addition to the use of a Doppler stethoscope or monitor for evaluating fetal status, the nurse may also use a Doppler instrument to monitor blood flow in patients who have altered arterial circulation. A portable Doppler instrument is about the size of a tissue box. A small flat transducer is placed over the vessel to be assessed, and when the unit is turned on, transmitted sound waves are bounced off the moving blood, producing a pulse heard via earphones. The portable Doppler unit also is very useful in the first few days after an arterial graft to assess the continued patency of the graft. It may also be used in a clinic setting to assess patients with chronic perfusion problems. The Doppler unit is sometimes used to monitor the blood pressure in shock when the blood pressure is barely audible. Pulses can be detected with the Doppler unit when the pulse is too faint to be felt with the fingertips (Phipps, 1979).

POSSIBLE RISKS FROM ULTRASOUND

There are two known effects of ultrasound in tissue: the production of heat and cavitation (Taylor & Dyson, 1980). Cavitation is the appearance of gas-filled bubbles in a sound field. Ultrasound waves over 100,000 Hz cause formation of gas bubbles in bacterial cells, killing the bacteria (French, 1980). As far as is known, the low-intensity dose of ultrasound used for sonograms is harmless to humans; there is no heat formation or cavitation in the tissues. The sound waves are delivered intermittently for sonograms and not continuously as with therapy.

Sonograms have been used in pregnancy since the mid-1960s, and there have not been any reports of any damage to either the woman or the fetus (American College of Obstetricians and Gynecologists, 1979). Studies are continuing to determine if there are any possible long-term effects. The Doppler devices used in fetal monitoring are of low enough dosages to be free of adverse heating effects or cavitation in tissues. However, the Doppler instrument used in arterial studies does use intensities of sound that produce some heat in tissues; consequently, arterial Doppler monitors are not considered suitable for fetal investigation (Taylor & Dyson, 1980). Certainly, there is no risk of radiation with the ultrasound scan, as there is with radionuclide scans or x-rays. Thus, ultrasound may be frequently used without concern of radiation effects. In fact it is very rare to see fetal x-rays done anymore because of the radiation hazard. (See Chapter 1 on pregnancy and radiation.)

PELVIC SONOGRAMS: ULTRASOUND SCANS IN PREGNANCY AND GYNECOLOGIC CONDITIONS

Purposes: As mentioned earlier, sonograms were originally used for evaluating the position of the placenta and the status of the fetus. Before an amniocentesis (Chapter 9) is done the position of the placenta is determined by ultrasound. The fetal growth rate can also be determined by measurements of the pictures taken by ultrasound. Ectopic pregnancies, hydatidiform moles, or structural abnormalities in the fetus can all be detected by ultrasound. The presence of twins can almost always be detected, too. It is possible, however, for one twin to "hide" behind the other so that the two-dimensional scan does not show the second fetus. In questionable scans, several sonograms may be done. One of the great advantages of ultrasound is that repeated scans are not risky. If necessary, sonograms may be done several times during a pregnancy. Ultrasound scans may also be done after a delivery to check for any retained placenta. Pelvic sonograms are also used to evaluate pelvic inflammatory disease and abscess formation. Pelvic masses can also be detected with ultrasound. The use of ultrasound in pregnancy and gynecologic conditions is a very sophisticated art, and numerous articles and books have been written on the subject. Sanders (1980) describes in detail the usefulness of ultrasound in diagnosing fetal death.

Pretest Nursing Implications for Pregnant Women

The movement of the transducer over the abdomen is not at all painful. The patient can see the scan on the monitor. Most pregnant women are thrilled to be able to see a picture of the baby on the monitoring screen. The technician can point out the head, feet, etc. of the baby as it moves about. The heart beat is seen as a blip of light. At Children's Hospital in San Francisco, any woman who wishes a picture of her baby is given a copy of the sonogram. Obviously, watching the monitor can be an unbelievable, chilling moment for the woman whose child is dead or if the ultrasound is being done to assess malformations.

Besides the anxiety of finding possible abnormalities with the sonogram, two other factors may make a sonogram slightly uncomfortable for the pregnant woman. One factor is the need for the woman to have a full bladder during the procedure. A full bladder is an "acoustical window" so that other structures can be seen in relation to the bladder. Sound waves travel well through liquid. The other factor is the need for the woman to lie in a flat position for twenty or so minutes. Some pregnant women can get hypotensive from the pressure on the vena cava. It may be necessary for the woman to turn on her left side to relieve this pressure.

Physical Preparations Before All Pelvic Sonograms

There is no need to restrict any medications nor alter the patient's diet before the test. It is essential, however, that the patient's bladder be full during the sonogram; thus, the patient must drink about ¾ quart of water (750 ml) before the test. As noted above, a full bladder

TABLE 7. PREPARATION OF PATIENT FOR SONOGRAPHY

Test	N.P.O.?	Bowel Prep?	Other
Pelvic sonograms	No	No	Must have full bladder
Abdominal sonograms	Usually but not always	Varies	See text for medication used and other prep
Echocardiograms	No	No	None
Echoencephalograms	No	No	Sedation for children?
Thoracic sonograms	No	No	None

is an "acoustical window." If the patient has an intravenous going, the nurse needs to check to see how much the IV rate should be increased. If the patient has a Foley catheter, the catheter must be clamped so that the bladder is full for the pelvic sonogram. (See Table 7.) As with the pregnant woman, but to a lesser degree, the discomfort of maintaining a full bladder for the time of the test is expected.

Posttest Nursing Implications

There are no special nursing implications after the patient has had a pelvic sonogram. If the sonogram was done to assess for fetal abnormalities or fetal death (demise), the nurse should know. This will be a very sad time for the patient. The nurse must be sensitive, helping the woman find the needed support to cope with the distressing news. (See Chapter 9 for a discussion on the role of the nurse in helping couples deal with loss.)

ABDOMINAL SONOGRAMS

Purposes: Sonography of the abdomen is being used more and more as the equipment becomes more sophisticated and clinicians become more adept at identifying abdominal problems by sonogram. A sonogram of the abdomen may mean the patient does not need to have exposure to radiation or invasive procedures done to diagnose a problem.

Sometimes surgery can be avoided if sonograms are done. For example, sonograms of a dilated biliary tree can be used to differentiate between intrahepatic and extrahepatic obstruction with 96 percent accuracy (Taylor et al., 1979). An extrahepatic obstruction requires surgery, but an intrahepatic obstruction does not. Whalen (1979) contains a series of ten flow charts that show how ultrasound can be used to help diagnose ten common abdominal problems. These ten common abdominal problems are:

1. Retroperitoneal adenopathy
2. Aortic aneurysm
3. Renal mass
4. Nonfunctioning kidney
5. Adrenal mass
6. Pancreatic mass
7. Liver mass

8. Obstructive jaundice
9. Acute cholecystitis
10. Chronic cholecystitis or gallstones

For the diagnosis of some of these abdominal conditions, ultrasound may be the first test performed. In other clinical conditions, abdominal sonograms are complementary to other work-ups, such as radionuclide studies (Chapter 3) and x-ray studies (Chapter 1) or CT scans (Chapter 2). Various studies, such as Snow et al. (1979), have compared the usefulness of scintigraphy (radionuclides), sonography, and computer tomography (CT) for various types of abdominal pathology. In addition to no radiation hazard, sonography has the advantage of being less costly than methods using radionuclides or x-rays.

Pretest Nursing Implications

The actual procedure for an abdominal sonogram is similar to that of a pelvic sonogram, discussed earlier. However, the patient does not need to have a full bladder for an abdominal sonogram as for a pelvic sonogram. The patient may be on n.p.o. status or may be allowed only liquids, depending on the exact nature of the abdominal sonogram. For example, if the gallbladder is the focus, the patient will need to be on n.p.o. status for 12 hours. If the patient eats before the sonogram of the gallbladder, the gallbladder will be less full and thus not as easily visualized. For other scans, the purpose of allowing only liquids is to reduce gas formation in the colon because it may interfere with the scan. Another way to reduce gas in the gastrointestinal tract is by administering drugs with simethicon (Mylicon). Smoking and gum chewing are prohibited because they increase gas formation. Sometimes an enema is needed to clear the bowel. (See Chapter 1 for principles of bowel preps.) Abdominal scars and obesity make it difficult to obtain a good abdominal sonogram. Abdominal dressings must be removed before the sonogram. If the scan is a static scan, the patient will need to hold his or her breath for 20 seconds at a time so the diaphragm will be static. (See the earlier discussion on use of real-time imaging versus static scans.) Children should be given a chance to practice holding their breath before the scan is begun. Even young children can cooperate if they are not overly anxious and they are told to hold their breath while the assistant counts to 20. (See Chapter 6 on preparing children for diagnostic procedures.)

Posttest Nursing Implications

The patient may be ill from the underlying pathophysiology that necessitated the sonogram, but there is no concern over the direct effects of a sonogram. Occasionally, the sonogram may only be a preliminary test to some invasive procedure, such as a liver or renal biopsy. If so, the invasive procedure will have some direct nursing implications (see Chapter 6).

ECHOCARDIOGRAMS

Purposes: Ultrasound has become a well-established diagnostic tool for valvular defects. Ultrasound was first used to detect abnormalities in the mitral valve. The echocardiogram is also used to measure the diameters of the cardiac chambers and evaluate other structural abnormalities of the heart. Pleural effusion and cardiac tamponade are other abnormalities identified by ultrasound (Disch, 1980). Earlier echos used the M mode (motion) to do time motion studies of the heart. Newer types can also do cross-sectional scans, which can detect some changes in coronary vessels. However, at the present time, myocardial infarction cannot be assessed with an echocardiogram (Wenger et al., 1980). Thallium scanning (Chapter 3) shows promise as a radionuclide scanning of the heart for infarcted areas.

Pretest Nursing Implications

The patient needs no special preparation. The echocardiology technician will direct the beam of ultrasound at specific points on the patient's chest to get pictures of the mitral valve, etc. During the test the patient may be asked to do the Valsalva maneuver. Also, the patient may be given a vasodilator, such as amyl nitrate, that can have a side effect of tachycardia.

Posttest Nursing Implications

There is no specific care of the patient after an echocardiogram because it is a noninvasive procedure.

ECHOENCEPHALOGRAMS

Purposes: Ultrasonic visualizations of the head may be used to evaluate certain head injuries, including the initial stages of stroke. Computerized tomography (CT scan) is much more valuable in identifying masses and tumors because the CT scan is a three-dimensional cross section of the entire head (see Chapter 2). However, echoencephalograms are safe, have a relatively low cost, and can be done in special care units. They are effective to monitor certain cerebral pathologies. For example, ultrasound has been useful in monitoring the state of hydrocephalus in young infants. The size of the ventricles and the functions of the shunts are monitored by echoencephalograms or echoventriculograms (Babcock et al., 1980). In newborn infants, ultrasound can be used to assess for intracranial hemorrhages.

Pretest Nursing Implications

As with other ultrasound procedures, there is no pain or risk for the patient. The head is placed on a foam sponge. If the echoencephalogram is done on a small child, the nurse may need to hold the child's head. Then, a water soluble gel is applied to the skull. Thick hair may make it difficult to do a sonogram, but any cutting of the hair must be done via hospital procedure. During the sonogram the patient must remain motionless. If the patient cannot lie still during the exam, the physician may order a sedative. Drugs, food, and fluids can be taken normally. Portable ultrasound units may be wheeled to neurologic units or newborn nurseries to avoid transporting critically ill patients.

Posttest Nursing Implications

There is no special aftercare, but the nurse should be aware of underlying pathophysiology, which may indicate a need for frequent neurologic assessments. The patient may wish to wash his or her hair to remove the gel.

THORACIC SONOGRAMS

Purposes: Because ultrasound does not penetrate air, sonograms are not as useful for thoracic disease as for abdominal disease. In order for a lesion to be identified by ultrasound, there must be no air-filled lung between the chest wall and the lesion. Sonograms of the chest may be useful in identifying pleural fluid, abscess formation, or malposition of the diaphragm (Spitz, 1980).

Nursing Implications

There is no special preparation of the patient and no special care after the procedure.

Questions

1. Sonograms or ultrasound scans are done with ultrasound waves, which are

a. Waves of energy closely related to the gamma rays of x-ray
b. High frequency sound waves, which are beyond the range of audible sound
c. Sound waves of very low frequency that are undetectable by the human ear
d. Part of a still undefined physical force

2. The type of ultrasound scan that demonstrates motion, such as the movement of a fetus is

a. A mode scan **b.** B scan **c.** Real-time scan **d.** Doppler scan

3. The nurse may use the Doppler method of ultrasound to assess all these patients except

a. Mrs. Jarvis, who is in the first stage of labor
b. Mr. Bixby, who has had an aortic-femoral bypass
c. Mr. Tucker, who had a pacemaker inserted yesterday
d. Mrs. Horn, who is undergoing an oxyctocin challenge test (OCT)

4. One of the known physical effects of *large continuous* doses of ultrasound is

a. Decreased circulation to the body part
b. Generation of heat in the body part
c. Radiation burn in deep tissues
d. Skin breakdown and redness in superficial layers

5. Which of the following is essential preparation before a *pelvic* sonogram? The patient must

a. Maintain n.p.o. status
b. Be given an enema or suppository
c. Not take any medications
d. Have a full bladder

6. Which of the following preparations is not necessary when the patient is having an *abdominal* sonogram?

a. Removing abdominal dressings
b. No smoking for several hours before the exam
c. Use of drugs such as simethicone for antiflatulent activity
d. Having the patient drink two to three glasses of water before the exam

7. Echocardiograms are useful diagnostic tools for detecting all but

a. Valvular defects
b. Cardiac tamponade
c. Pleural effusion
d. Myocardial infarction

8. Baby Dabney is having an echoencephalogram done to monitor a ventricular shunt that was inserted for hydrocephalus. The responsibilities of the nurse who accompanies the baby to the ultrasound department may include all *except*

a. Explaining the results of the sonogram to the parents
b. Reassuring the mother that the exam is not painful for the child
c. Giving an ordered sedative before the exam
d. Holding the baby's head while the sonogram is being done

9. The use of ultrasound in the thorax is severely limited because

a. The transducer cannot be moved evenly on the chest wall.
b. Ultrasound does not penetrate air.
c. Thoracic tumors are solid masses.
d. The movement of the heart interferes with the sound waves.

REFERENCES

American College of Obstetricians and Gynecologists, Committee on Patient Education. *Ultrasound Examinations in OB-Gyn*. Chicago: 1979.

Babcock, D. et al. "B-Mode Gray Scale Ultrasound of the Head in the Newborn and Young Infant." *American Journal of Roentgenology* 134: 457–468 (March 1980).

Disch, J. *Diagnostic Procedures for Cardiovascular Disease*. Norwalk, CT: Appleton-Century-Crofts, 1980.

French, R. *Guide to Diagnostic Procedures*. New York: McGraw-Hill, 1980.

James, E. "Future Developments in Ultrasound." In *Principles and Practices of Ultrasound in Obstetrics and Gynecology*, 2nd ed. (Roger Sanders, ed.) Norwalk, CT: Appleton-Century-Crofts, 1980.

Kreel, L. & Steiner, R., eds. Section 6, "Ultrasonography" *Medical Imaging*. Chicago: Year Book Medical Publishers, Inc., 1979.

Meire, H. B. "Ultrasound—Current Status and Prospects." *British Journal of Radiology* 50: 379–380 (June 1977).

Phipps, W., et al. *Medical Surgical Nursing: Concepts and Clinical Practice*. St. Louis: C. V. Mosby, 1979.

Pachaczevsk, R. ''Simple Transducer Supported Water Bath Device for Ultrasonography.'' *American Journal of Roentgenology* 133: 553–555 (September 1979).

''Research Roundup.'' *UCSF Magazine* 3: 29 (March 1980).

Sanders, R. ''Ultrasound in the Diagnosis of Fetal Death'' In *Principles and Practices of Ultrasonography in Obstetrics and Gynecology,* 2nd ed. (Roger Sanders, ed.) Norwalk, CT: Appleton-Century-Crofts, 1980.

Snow, J. et al. ''Comparisons of Scintigraphy, Sonography and Computed Tomography in the Evaluation of Hepatic Neoplasma.'' *American Journal of Roentgenology* 132: 915–917 (June 1979).

Spitz, H. ''Use of Ultrasound in the Thorax.'' *Basics of Respiratory Disease* 9: 5 (September 1980).

Taylor, K. et al. ''Diagnostic Accuracy of Gray Scale Ultrasonography for the Jaundiced Patient.'' *Archives of Internal Medicine* 139: 60–63 (January 1979).

Taylor, K. & Dyson, M. ''Experimental Insonation of Animal Tissues and Fetuses.'' In *Principles and Practices of Ultrasonography in Obstetrics and Gynecology,* 2nd ed. (Roger Sanders, ed.) Norwalk, CT: Appleton-Century-Crofts, 1980.

Whalen, J. ''Newer Imaging Methods of the Abdomen.'' *American Journal of Roentgenology* 133: 587–615 (October 1979).

Wells, P. ''Ultrasound Limits, Resolution and Equipment.'' In *Medical Imaging* (Kreel, K., ed.) Chicago: Year Book Medical Publishers, Inc., 1979.

Wenger, N. et al. *Cardiology for Nurses*. New York: McGraw-Hill, 1980.

Ziskin, M. ''Basic Principles of Ultrasound.'' In *Principles and Practices of Ultrasonography in Obstetrics and Gynecology* (Roger Sanders, ed.) Norwalk, CT: Appleton-Century-Crofts, 1980.

CHAPTER FIVE

Common Noninvasive Diagnostic Tests

Objectives

1. Describe the usual role of the nurse in preparing patients for noninvasive diagnostic testing.
2. Describe five basic characteristics of a normal sinus rhythm on a Lead II ECG strip and how common arrhythmias change these characteristics.
3. Given an ECG of a normal sinus rhythm, calculate the heart rate of the patient.
4. State what nursing assessments are useful in monitoring the mechanical events of the heart when the patient has an abnormal ECG or is on telemetry.
5. Compare the uses and techniques of vectorcardiograms, phonocardiograms, and ballistograms as three noninvasive measures of cardiac function.
6. State four important nursing functions to help prepare a patient for an EEG.
7. Describe what a nurse should teach a patient about an EMG.
8. Explain how the pulmonary function tests, FVC, FEV, MVV, and FEF are used in assessing lung ventilation defects that are obstructive or restrictive.
9. Describe how the measurement of heat is accomplished with diagnostic thermography.

The preceding four chapters covered specific types of noninvasive procedures, which use x-rays (Chapters 1 and 2), radionuclides (Chapter 3), and ultrasound (Chapter 4). This chapter covers several types of noninvasive tests, including measuring such diverse things as electric events (ECG, EEG, and EMG), audible sound (phonocardiogram), projectile forces (ballistocardiograph), air flow (pulmonary function tests), and body surface heat (thermography) (see Table 8). The unifying theme throughout all of these tests is: because they are noninvasive, there is little or no risk to the patient. These tests give an indirect assessment of an organ and its structure or function. Most are fairly easy to perform (usually done by a skilled technician) and are relatively inexpensive.

TABLE 8. NONINVASIVE DIAGNOSTIC PROCEDURES USING VARIOUS TYPES OF MEASUREMENTS[a]

	Electrical Event	Sound	Ultrasound[b]	Force	Air Flow	Heat	X-Rays[c]
Heart	ECG Vectorgrams Telemetry Holter monitors	Phonocardiogram	Echocardiogram	Ballistogram			Chest x-rays
Brain	EEG		Encephalogram				Skull films CT scan
Muscles	EMG						
Lungs			Thoracic sonogram		Spirometry		Chest x-rays Tomogram CT scan
Tumors or Inflammation			Abdominal and pelvic sonograms			Thermography	Flat plates of abdomen CT Scan

[a] *See this chapter for general nursing implications for noninvasive diagnostic testing.*
[b] *See Chapter 4.*
[c] *See Chapters 1 and 2.*

Invasive diagnostic tests are those that utilize methods that invade the body, such as cardiac catheterization (Chapter 7) or an endoscopy procedure (Chapter 8). Other common invasive procedures are the subject of Chapter 6. The nurse must realize that this division of invasive and noninvasive tests is strictly from the professional's view. For the patient, *any* test is an invasion of his or her personal space and privacy. Although the health professional considers an ECG noninvasive (because the body is not entered), the patient may (because of the use of electrodes on his or her body) perceive it as being very invasive. The same holds true for the use of needles with an EMG, even though the invasion is under the skin and not into the body proper.

GENERAL NURSING IMPLICATIONS

Pretest

It is the nurse's responsibility to see that the patient is both physically and psychologically ready for the test. Preparation of the patient should include reassurance that the test is neither painful nor harmful. Note that pain from the needles used for EMG (and sometimes EEG) is momentary and does not require a local anesthetic, as do the tests covered in the next chapter. Special consent forms are not needed because there is no anticipation of any complications from the test itself. There are very specific physical preparations for several of the tests, such as a shampoo before an EEG. Certain drugs affect the results of several of these tests; thus, the nurse must be aware of what information needs to be put on laboratory requests. Also, the nurse must make sure the patient understands any restrictions on drugs, food, or liquids.

Posttest

With a few exceptions, there are no specific nursing implications after noninvasive testing. Although these tests are relatively simple to perform and there is practically no risk to the patient, the patient may be quite ill from their basic pathologic problem. The aftercare of the patient is therefore geared to the underlying problems. The general focus of nursing care after a noninvasive test is to let the patient rest once an assessment has been done. It is important for the nurse to validate that the patient is physically stable and not psychologically upset by the test, which was done. The results of the test may not be known for a while, and this may be a source of anxiety for the patient. (See the discussion in Chapter 1 on posttest anxiety.)

ELECTROCARDIOGRAMS

Description: An electrocardiogram (ECG or EKG) comprises the electrical impulses generated by the heart during its depolarization and repolarization that are picked up by electrodes and are displayed on a strip of graph paper. These electrodes are fastened to all four of the patient's extremities by rubber straps. A jelly or paste is used under each electrode to help conduction of the electric impulse. The electrodes on both arms and the left leg are used to record impulses. The electrode on the right leg is just a ground. A suction bulb is moved across the patient's chest to obtain six different views of the heart (precordial leads).

The most common lead used for monitoring (and the one usually displayed in nursing textbooks) is Lead II, which records the electric activity of the heart by using the negative electrode on the right arm and the positive electrode on the left leg. As the heart's electric current moves down through the heart, the current moving toward the positive electrode will show as a positive deflection on the graph (above the baseline). If the electric current moves away from the positive electrode, the graph will show a negative deflection (below the baseline). In Lead II, as the electric current goes down through the atrium and the ventricles, there are two positive deflections: P-wave and QRS complex. In other leads, such as the augmented leads, the P-wave and QRS complex will be seen as negative deflections because of the placement of the electrodes. Lead I uses both arm electrodes and Lead III uses the left arm and left leg electrodes. In addition to these three leads (I, II, and III) and the six precordial leads (V_1 through V_6), there are also three augmented unipolar leads (a VR, a VL, and a VF), which make up the standard 12-lead electrocardiogram. Six inches of each lead are taken. With all 12 leads of the ECG, a clinician can gain a great deal of knowledge about the total electric activity of the heart. However, for basic monitoring of the patient or for an assessment of an arrhythmia, Lead II may suffice.

Purposes: The ECG is a diagnostic tool used very frequently for patients with chest pain or other cardiac symptoms. The ECG is the definitive way to diagnose the various arrhythmias. It is also very helpful in distinguishing myocardial infarction from myocardial ischemia. A cardiologist interprets the ECG and writes a formal summary of his or her findings. This summary is put in the chart with samples from the various leads of the ECG.

Characteristics of a Normal Sinus Rhythm

Although the formal interpretation of the ECG is done by a cardiologist, the nurse should have some understanding of what a normal sinus rhythm (NSR) looks like (see Figure 1). The characteristics of a normal ECG are (Wenger et al., 1980):

1. The heart rate is between 60 and 100 in an adult (two ways to calculate rates are discussed later).
2. The rhythm is regular.
3. A P-wave precedes each QRS complex.
4. The P–R interval is between 0.12 and 0.20 seconds.
5. The QRS complex is normal and less than 0.10 seconds.
6. The T-wave is normal.

Describing Arrhythmias

In describing arrhythmias, a normal *sinus* rhythm (NSR) means that the heart rate is under the control of the sino-atrial node (SA node). A *sinus* tachycardia means that the rate is faster than 100, in the adult, but the SA node is still controlling the rate. On the other hand, *atrial* tachycardia means that the atrium is controlling the heart rate, whereas a

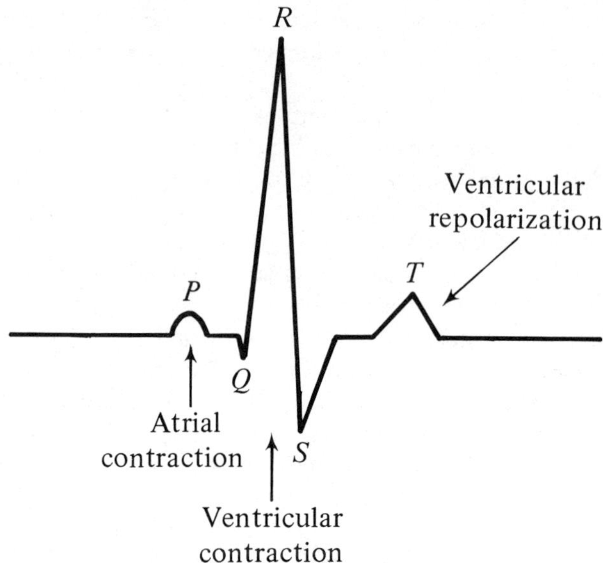

Figure 1. Basic components of an ECG tracing. (Note that atrial repolarization is hidden in QRS complex.) See text for definition of: P–wave; P–R interval; QRS complex; T–wave; Q–T intervals; S–T segment.

ventricular tachycardia means that the ventricle is controlling the heart rate. In *nodal* or junctional arrhythmias, the A–V node is controlling the rate. Thus, by just reading the name of the arrhythmia from the ECG report, the nurse can assess something about the origin of the arrhythmia.

Ectopic or Premature Beats

A premature ventricular contraction (PVC) occurs when the ventricle originates a beat before the normal conduction of the impulse from the SA node. In rhythms with an occasional premature beat, the cardiac rate is still being controlled by the SA node. Another name for premature beats is ectopic beats, which means displaced or malpositioned. (An ectopic pregnancy occurs outside the uterus.) Ectopic or premature contractions can arise from the atrial tissue (PAC), ventricular tissue (PVC), or from A–V junctional tissue. Vaz (1979) includes examples of all of the common cardiac arrhythmias, as do most nursing texts (see for example Phipps et al., 1979; Luckmann & Sorensen, 1980).

P-Wave

The P-wave occurs at the beginning of each contraction of the atria (depolarization). The rounded P-wave is the impulse spreading through muscle, not going down conductive tissue in a straight line. (In contrast, the QRS complex is a straight line with a peak because the impulse is traveling directly down conductive tissue.)

Abnormal P-Wave

In premature atrial contraction (PAC), the P-wave will look different, not the usual sequence seen with the normal sinus rhythm. In arrhythmias, such as atrial fibrillation, the P-waves cannot be distinguished on the ECG because the atria are quivering or fibrillating. In atrial enlargement, the P-wave will look different because the impulse travels through more tissue.

P–R Interval

The P–R interval is the time it takes the impulse to travel from the atrium to the ventricle through the AV node and the Bundle of His. Normally the P–R interval in 0.12 to 0.20 second. (One large square on the ECG paper measures 0.20 second.)

A P–R interval longer than 0.20 second indicates a slowing of the impulse through the AV node and Bundle of His. Drugs, such as digitalis, can cause a widening P–R interval or first degree heart block. Other types of drugs may also prolong the P–R interval. In one type of second degree heart block, the P–R interval gets longer and longer until the ventricular beat is dropped. In a complete heart block, the P–R interval cannot be measured because the ventricles are originating beats that are totally independent of the SA impulses, which generate the atrial beats. Thus, in complete heart block, the P-waves may be normal, but no QRS complex follows. The P-waves and QRS complexes will be totally independent of each other.

QRS Complex

The QRS complex reflects the contraction (depolarization) of the ventricles. Normally, the QRS complex is less than .12 second.

An ectopic beat, which arises from the ventricle (PVC), will cause a distorted and widened QRS complex. A PVC usually looks very different from the other QRS complexes in the strip. Often, the QRS complex will be a negative deflection rather than the positive deflection seen in Lead II. All of these changes in the QRS complex are due to an impulse that originated in ventricular tissue and traveled through the ventricle differently than the normal impulse, which comes from the SA node.

In myocardial infarction, the appearance of the QRS complex is one part of the ECG that is changed. Abnormal Q-waves are characteristic of myocardial infarction, but other conditions can cause changes in the Q-waves, too (Luckmann & Sorensen, 1980).

In ventricular tachycardia, the ventricles have taken control of the heart rate, and the ECG shows only spikes of QRS complexes, which are wide and rather bizarre looking.

ECG Documentation of the Type of Cardiac Arrest

In ventricular fibrillation, there are only wavy lines on the ECG with nothing that resembles a P-wave or QRS complex. Ventricular fibrillation causes cardiac arrest—when the ventricles are fibrillating (quivering) there is no cardiac output—and the ECG shows chaotic electric activity. For the other type of cardiac arrest, cardiac standstill or asystole, the ECG shows a straight line—even the quivering or fibrillation of the ventricle has stopped. Only the ECG can distinguish whether a cardiac arrest is due to asystole or fibrillation.

T-Wave

The T-wave occurs as the ventricles recover from the contraction period. This period of electrical recovery is called repolarization. (The repolarization of the atrium is not seen on the ECG graph because it is hidden in the larger electrical event of the QRS complex.)

Myocardial damage may cause inversion of the T-waves. High levels of serum potassium (hyperkalemia) cause tall, peaked T-waves. An ECG on an oscilloscope is sometimes used to monitor potassium replacement in severe cases of hypokalemia. Low levels of potassium (hypokalemia) cause inverted T-waves. A flattened T-wave means the ventricle is not able to repolarize normally.

Q–T Interval

The Q–T interval covers the period of both ventricular depolarization and repolarization. Its normal duration is 0.36 to 0.44 second.

The Q–T interval is useful in evaluating the effects of drugs on the heart, such as quinidine. Ischemia or electrolyte changes may prolong or shorten the Q–T interval.

S–T Segment

The S–T segment is the time between completion of depolarization and the beginning of repolarization of the ventricles. One often interpretes only a nonspecific S–T abnormality on an ECG.

A decidely depressed or downward slope of the S–T segment is somewhat characteristic of myocardial ischemia. Digitalis will cause depression of the S–T segment, as well. (See the "Stress Test" in Chapter 7 for more explanation about S–T changes from exertion and other factors.) Conversely, an elevated S–T segment is one of the characteristics of a myocardial infarction. As with all other changes in the ECG, the meaning of the changes may be open to several interpretations, depending on other clinical data.

DETERMINING PULSE RATE WITH AN ECG

Because the ECG paper is horizontally marked for time, pulse rate can be determined by looking at an ECG strip. (The vertical deflections reflect the amplitude of the voltage, but this is not of major usefulness to the nurse who is just beginning to learn about ECGs.) As seen in Figure 2, each tiny square of ECG strip measures 0.04 second, and each larger square (which consists of five tiny ones) is 0.20 second. By remembering that each large square signifies a time of 0.20 second, one can calculate the pulse rate by several different formulas. Two simple methods that a nurse can use to time a pulse rate by scanning an ECG strip are discussed below. Both of these methods assume a steady rate of impulses.

Method A: Counting the Squares between the Beats

The squares between each QRS complex can be counted to determine the time between each beat. For example, if there are three large squares between each beat (QRS complex), this implies a time interval of (3 squares $\times$ 0.2 second) 0.6 second between each beat. Thus, in 60 seconds, there would be (60 seconds divided by 0.6) 100 beats. If there were five large squares between each beat, this would mean (5 $\times$ 0.20 second) 1 second

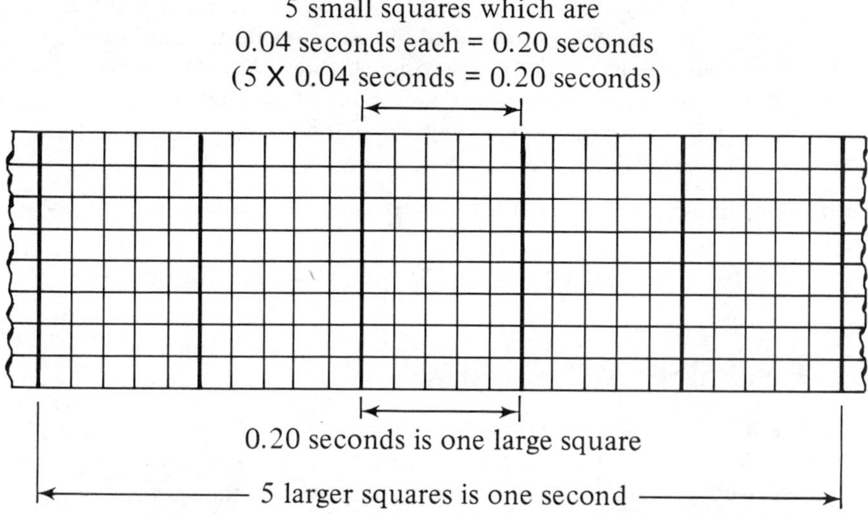

Figure 2. Two methods to determine pulse rate from an ECG tracing.

Method A: Count the number of large squares that occur between each QRS complex.

Formula: $\dfrac{\text{60 Seconds}}{\text{Number of Squares between Beats} \times \text{0.2 second}} = \text{Beats per Minute}$

Method B: Count the number of beats in 30 large squares.

Formula: Number of Beats in 30 Squares $\times$ 10 = Beats per Minute

*See text for examples of use.

between each beat. In 60 seconds, there would be (60 seconds divided by 1 second per beat) 60 beats. Thus, when a patient has a normal rhythm on an ECG strip, which has no fewer than three squares and no more than five squares between beats, the rate is within the normal adult range of 60 to 100 beats per minute, respectively. The formula for calculating pulse rate by this method is:

$$\frac{\text{60 Seconds per Minute}}{\text{Number of squares between Beats} \times \text{0.20 Seconds}} = \text{Beats per Minute.}$$

Example:

$$\frac{60}{\text{30 (Squares between Beats)} \times 0.20} = \frac{60}{0.6} = 100.$$

Method B: Counting the Beats in 30 Squares

Another way to calculate the heart rate from an ECG strip is to count the number of QRS complexes in a certain number of squares. Recall that the large square measures 0.20 second in time. By counting the beats in 30 large squares, one has counted the number of beats occuring in six seconds because 30 squares × 0.20 second equals six seconds. The number obtained for six seconds is multiplied by ten to obtain the number of beats per minute. The time markings on the ECG strip designate three-second intervals and can also be used to determine six-second segments. For example, if the total number of beats in 30 squares is five, then the pulse rate is 50 (five beats in 0.6 second × 10). The formula for this method of calculating pulse rate is:

Number of Beats in 30 Squares (or 0.6 Seconds) × 10 = Number of Beats per Minute
Example:

5 Beats (in 30 Squares) × 10 = 50 Beats per Minute

PRETEST NURSING IMPLICATIONS

Because many drugs, such as quinidine or digitalis, affect certain aspects of the ECG, it is important that the cardiologist who interprets the test be aware of any cardiac drugs the patient has received. Most ECG requests have a place to note the cardiac drugs that the patient has received.

It is not necessary to withhold drugs or food from the patient before an ECG. The patient should not wear metal jewelry. Clothing must be loose so the electrodes can be fastened on the arms and legs and the suction bulb moved across the chest. Women will need to remove hose because the electrode paste must be applied directly to the skin. The jelly or paste used with the electrodes is nonallergic, but it may feel messy to the patient. Patients may be slightly skeptical about "being strapped to an electrical box," as a patient once said. Therefore, the patient may need reassurance that the machine only detects electrical signals *from* the patient and not to the patient.

Tips on Electrical Safety

From a safety point of view, any electrical equipment does have the potential for an electrical hazard if the machine is defective and not properly grounded. As a general rule, all electrically operated appliances for a patient should be plugged into the same wall outlet so there is no difference in ground points. Improperly grounded or defective equipment can cause a current leakage through the patient if the two pieces of equipment are plugged into outlets more than 12 feet apart (Meth, 1980). The ECG technician has the responsibility of checking the machine to make sure that there are no frayed cords, etc., and that the machine is properly grounded. The nurse just needs to keep in mind that for very ill patients, such as those with electrodes placed into the ventricle, all electrical equipment must be checked and grounded properly, including ECG machines. The nurse should consult with the hospital's electrical engineer about any problems that occur and how to do safety checks of routine equipment.

POSTTEST NURSING IMPLICATIONS

The ECG technician helps the patient wipe off the electrode paste or jelly. Aside from this, there is no other special patient care related directly to the test in general. However, if the ECG was done to evaluate a possible myocardial infarction, cardiac precautions should be continued until other diagnostic tests, such as cardiac enzymes, are interpreted by the patient's physician. If the ECG was done to evaluate an arrhythmia, the nurse may need to inquire about any changes in medication orders. Usually the ECG technician scans the graph for blatant abnormalities and calls this to the attention of the physician. Sometimes the ECG strip is kept with the patient's chart; thus, the patient's personal physician can immediately evaluate the strip. Otherwise the interpretation of the ECG will be done by a cardiologist, and a typed summary will later appear on the patient's chart.

Assessing the Mechanical Events of the Heart

Heart rate, rhythm, and the presence or absence of a pulse deficit should be routinely monitored by the nurse if there is any question of arrhythmias. The nurse must remember that the ECG is measuring only the electrical events in the heart and not the cardiac output. Westfall (1976) describes, in detail, the many bedside assessments that the nurse can make, which measure the mechanical events of the heart.

Apart from assessing the ECG strip, the nurse should be aware of the signs of cardiac dysfunction. The quality of peripheral pulses, capillary filling time, and color of the patient are all signs of the adequacy or inadequacy of cardiac output. Noting any dyspnea, angina, abnormal heart or breath sounds, and a decrease in urine output are all determined by the nurse—not detected from an ECG reading. Therefore, even when the patient is on a monitor of the ECG pattern, the nurse must still collect the above information to obtain a complete picture of the efficiency of the heart.

VECTORCARDIOGRAM

A vectorgram and an ECG differ only in the type of instrument used to record and analyze the electrical events of the heart. A mathematical analysis of the different leads (usually six) is done to detect the direction and magnitude of electric energy on a moment-to-moment basis (Disch, 1980). The vectorgram gives a three-dimensional picture of the heart, which comprises a P loop, QRS loop, and ST–T segment loop. A vectorcardiogram may be very helpful in evaluating conduction defects or abnormal impulse pathways, which are not as evident on the conventional ECG. The patient can be told that a vectorgram is a "sophisticated" ECG. Otherwise, the nursing implications are the same as for the routine ECG.

DIAGNOSTIC MONITORING IN INTENSIVE CARE UNITS

Patients with the potential for serious cardiac arrhythmias may be connected to cardiac monitors, which provide continuous surveillance of the electrical impulses of the heart. The ECG pattern is displayed on an oscilloscope, and when needed, on graph paper for a permanent record. When the patient is connected to a monitor in an intensive care unit or coronary care unit, the nurse must have special training on how to recognize those arrhythmias that need immediate medical attention. Coronary care units may have standardized orders that permit a nurse, who has had special training, to administer antiarrhythmia drugs (such as lidocaine (Xylocaine), when the patient has certain patterns of premature ventricular contractions). Today's critical care nurse also focuses on early recognition of potentially lethal cardiac conduction defects by recognizing electric axis deviations on the ECG. Alspach (1979) is an example of the expanded role of the nurse in interpreting ECG readings. The reader is encouraged to consult one of the many excellent textbooks that focus on critical care nursing.

TELEMETRY

Telemetry is making measurements at a distance from the subject by the use of radio signals (Miller & Keane, 1978). Telemetry has been extensively used in assessing physiologic functioning during space travels. In the hospital setting, telemetry is used to monitor an ECG of a patient without the patient having to be hooked up to a monitor. Nurses on general care units may take care of a patient who is being monitored "long distance" by a monitor in the intensive care or coronary care unit. The critical care nurse monitors the monitor.

Small electrode discs are applied to the patient's chest to obtain a good reading on the monitor. Disposable prelubricated discs can be kept on the patient for several days unless skin irritation is noted. The wires from the electrodes are connected to a portable transmitter. The portable transmitter is about the size of a small tissue box, and can be left lying in bed by the patient or can be strapped to the ambulatory patient's waist. It should be reemphasized that telemetry, like a conventional ECG, only measures the rate and electrical events of the heart. The nurse is still needed to assess the mechanical events (i.e., cardiac output) of the patient. Westfall (1976) describes the role of the nurse when a patient on a general unit has telemetry.

Telemetry by Telephone

Telephone recordings of ECGs originated in 1971. A special instrument is used with the telephone. The heart rhythm's graphic representation is fed into a computer and a duplicate is made for analysis by a cardiologist. In San Francisco, the response time for emergency requests is from 10 to 15 minutes for a complete reading (Pacific Telephone Company, 1981). Patients with pacemakers may be followed by telephone.

AMBULATORY ECG RECORDING

In outpatient settings, patients may be given a portable recorder (sometimes referred to as Holter monitor) to wear, which records the ECG on magnetic tape. When the tapes are returned to the cardiology laboratory, a computer scans the tapes to pick out any specific points of interest. They are also evaluated by a physician. One brand name for a telephone heart monitor is Cardio Beeper[1] (Survival Technology, Bethesda, MD). This method is costly, but it can be very helpful in pinpointing the type of arrhythmia that is causing the

[1]See Streiff (1981) for a discussion on the usefullness of the Cardio Beeper for visiting nurses.

patient's symptoms. It can reduce the number of costly ambulance trips to the hospital. Also, the ambulatory ECG can be used to evaluate the effects of certain treatments. Nurses may prepare the patient for the test and scan the strips to see which patients need medical interventions.

Preparation of Patient for Ambulatory ECG Recording

The patient is not to swim or bathe when the monitor is in place. Also the patient must not have any x-rays while the monitor is being used—x-rays will erase the tape (Coats, 1975). The patient should be instructed to keep a diary of any events that cause such symptoms as shortness of breath, dizziness, or angina. The patient should also keep a record of such activities as sleeping time, exercise, or emotional stress, which may be related to the cardiac symptoms.

McNeal (1978), a nurse who works as a cardioscanalyst (the person inspecting the 24-hour strips), has observed that patients are often unaware that their symptoms, such as those discussed above, are due to an arrhythmia. In addition to the usual cardiac symptoms, symptoms such as headache, indigestion, or "feeling weak" may be linked to the specific time of an arrhythmia. Thus, a 24-hour strip may elucidate the cause of vague patient symptoms so that the symptoms can be treated.

Visiting nurses should instruct patients in the use of Holter monitors when it is necessary to evaluate arrhythmias related to physical reconditioning at home after cardiac surgery or postmyocardial infarction (Streiff, 1981).

PHONOCARDIOGRAMS

Description: The phonocardiogram is a graphic recording of the sounds generated during the cardiac cycle. The phonocardiogram is a sophisticated way to evaluate abnormal heart sounds, detected with a standard stethoscope. A microphone is positioned on the chest wall and picks up the sounds that are transmitted to the graph paper. The phonocardiogram is usually recorded in conjunction with an ECG, which records the electrical events of the heart, and a pulse tracing, which records the mechanical events of the heart.

Purpose: By documenting the precise time of the abnormal heart sound, in relation to the mechanical and electrical events of the heart, the cardiologist can better interpret the abnormal heart sound. (See echocardiograms, Chapter 4, on how sound waves are used for diagnosing heart problems.)

Nursing Implications

The patient can eat and have medications before the test. If the patient has a lot of hair on his chest, a small area may be shaved so that the microphone will not pick up the sounds from hair movement. During the test, the patient may be given vasodilating drugs, such as amyl nitrate, which can cause dizziness and light-headedness in some patients (Coats, 1975). Otherwise the test is not at all uncomfortable, and requires no special patient care afterward.

BALLISTOGRAMS

Ballistics is the study of motion and the impact of projectiles. A ballistogram is a record of the headward–footward movement of the body during the systolic ejection of blood. The patient is put on a special table, and the vibrations of the body are measured by a machine attached to the table. The ballistogram shows the force of the contraction of the heart and the force of the cardiac output. There is no discomfort to the patient, who just lies quietly on the table. The patient may feel the vibrations and be startled. There is no pre- or postcare for the patient (Allen, 1978).

ELECTROENCEPHALOGRAM (EEG)

Description: The electroencephalogram (EEG) is a recording of the brain's electrical activity. The EEG primarily records activity of the superficial layers of the cerebral cortex.

If the patient is comatose; the EEG can be done at his or her bedside. However, for routine diagnostic studies, the patient is taken to the EEG laboratory, where the environment can be better controlled. The recording takes an hour or two and includes a nap. The first part of the recording is done with the patient as relaxed as possible to obtain a baseline reading. The patient is then asked to hyperventilate for several minutes, to see how this changes the patterns of the brain. The patient may become a little light-headed from hyperventilating. The brain may also be stimulated by flickering lights. If the patient cannot nap for the last part of the test, a sedative, such as chloral hydrate, may be given (Shearer et al., 1975). Sleep may evoke abnormal patterns that are not present when the brain is more active.

Approximately 20 electrodes are applied to the patient's scalp. The electrode wires are attached to the EEG machine, which records the electric signals on a piece of graph paper. These electrodes may be surface electrodes or subdermal needle electrodes. The pain accompanying the subdermal needles is sometimes compared to the brief pain felt when one hair is pulled from the scalp. They are not very painful because the scalp is much less sensitive than other surface areas of the body. Most EEG laboratories use surface electrodes with a jelly to help conduction of the electric signals. The skin is wiped with acetone, and the area is slightly abraded with an electrical paste. It has been found that in children, this slight abrasion may cause calcium nodules in the skin (Wiley & Eaglstein, 1979). Thus, EEG paste with calcium chloride probably should not be used with young children or infants, whose skin has a less effective barrier against absorption of the calcium from the jelly. The papules of calcium do, however, disappear with no apparent harmful effects.

Purposes: Although the EEG is nonspecific, it can help identify a focus of disturbance in the brain. The majority of patients with cerebral seizures will have abnormal EEGs, but a normal EEG does not rule out a seizure disorder. About 10 percent of the patients with epilepsy have normal EEGs (Price & Wilson, 1978). The EEG must be correlated with other clinical assessments of the patient.

When the brain is dead, the electrical activity of the brain is absent, and the EEG is flat. The EEG is used as one of the ways to detect brain death in the comatose patient. In all the studies done on comatose patients, the findings of the EEG had a high correlation with the survival or death of the patient in a coma (Taylor & Ballenger, 1980).

Patient Preparation

For routine EEG testing, the patient should have no medicines for 24 to 48 hours before the test, except those medicines particularly ordered by the physician. Tranquilizers, stimulants (including coffee, tea, colas, and cigarettes), and alcohol all cause changes in brain patterns. The patient should have normal meals because hypoglycemia can also cause changes in brain patterns. The patient's hair should be shampooed the day before the test, and no oils, sprays, or lotions should be applied to the hair. It may be desirable that the patient not have much sleep before the EEG recording because sleep deprivation may evoke abnormal brain patterns. Also, as mentioned earlier, the last part of the EEG recording may be done with the patient asleep, and the patient may have trouble falling asleep if he or she has just had a lot of sleep. Therefore, the adult patient may be instructed to go to bed late the night before the test and to awake early. Children and infants should not be allowed to nap before the scheduled test.

If an EEG is being done to evaluate the possibility of brain death, it is important that artifacts be kept to a minimum. Artifacts can be caused by manipulation of the electrodes or by electrical interference. The nurse will need to follow the specific guidelines of the institution when EEGs are done at the patient's bedside (The electric hazards covered for the ECG would also be pertinent here where several electric applicances may be in use at once.)

Posttest Nursing Implications

The only specific care needed by the patient after an EEG is a shampoo to remove electrode gel from his or her hair. Also, as mentioned earlier, the calcium chloride in the gel may irritate the skin of children; thus, any gel on the skin must be carefully removed.

ELECTROMYELOGRAPH (EMG)

Description: The electromyelograph (EMG) measures the electrical activity of muscles. Needle electrodes are inserted into selected skeletal muscles. (Although in one sense the test is somewhat invasive, it is discussed here because of the similarities between ECGs and EMGs.) This procedure does cause some pain. The skin is cleansed with alcohol or iodine, but no local anesthetic is used. The muscle activity is recorded at rest, during voluntary activity, and with electric stimuli. The findings from the EMG are recorded and usually summarized in narrative form for use on the patient's chart.

Purposes: In nerve atrophy, there may be a characteristic fibrillation, even in the resting muscle. Usually a resting muscle has no electrical activity. The test can be useful in determining the extent of peripheral nerve injuries and differentiating paralysis of psychological origin.

The EMG cannot diagnose specific neuromuscular diseases, but it can specifically differentiate between neuropathy and myopathy (Spiegel, 1978). All neuromuscular abnormalities are classified in two categories:

1. *Myopathy* is a disease or disturbance of striated muscle fibers or cell membranes. Myasthenia gravis or primary muscular dystrophy are examples of myopathies that produce abnormal EMGs.
2. *Neuropathy* is a disease or disorder of the lower motor neuron. Toxic effects of drugs, hypothyroidism, polio, and diabetes can all cause neuropathy.

Nursing Implications

No special physical preparation of the patient is required before or after the test. Premedications for sedation or pain relief are avoided to assess a normal neuromuscular pattern (Ross, 1979). Muscle aches after the procedure may be relieved with mild analgesics. The procedure may take up to an hour or two if extensive testing is done. Before and after an EMG the nurse can be very useful in evaluating the functional capacity of the patient, with an unknown neuromuscular problem. Thus, the gait of the patient, ability to do ROM exercises, and any motor–power–sensory deficits should be recorded. Clinical data are always used as part of the base for interpreting EMG reports. Luckmann & Sorensen (1980) contains useful information on neuromuscular disorders and the nursing care needed. The nurse should prepare the patient for the discomfort and sounds of an EMG. The patient may feel pain on insertion of the needle electrodes and will hear audio amplification that sound like firecrackers (Bubb, 1982). If nerve conduction studies are done, the feelings may be similar to static electricity.

PULMONARY FUNCTION TESTS: SPIROMETRY

Description: Pulmonary function tests (PFT) can be classified as 1) ventilation tests and 2) specialized pulmonary function tests of gaseous diffusion and distribution. Pulmonary function tests, done in the pulmonary function laboratory, cover the entire range of respiratory volume and capabilities. On the other hand, pulmonary function tests done on the unit or in ambulatory care settings are modified to ventilation tests of FEV, VC, and MVV measures. This section focuses only on the more common ventilation studies. Chapter 3 includes information about lung perfusion scans. The clinical significance of blood gas analysis, an important aspect of many pulmonary studies, can be found in books on clinical laboratory tests such as Corbett (1982).

For ventilation studies of lung volume and capacity, the patient breathes into a machine called a spirometer. (The nurse sometimes uses a portable spirometer, the Wright spirometer, for clinical assessment of the patient's ventilation status.)

Purposes: Pulmonary function tests for lung volume and capacity help identify whether the patient has an obstructive defect, a restrictive defect, or a combination of both (Boyce & King, 1980). When there is an increase in airway resistance, the defect in ventilation is called an *obstructive defect*. Asthma, bronchitis, and emphysema cause obstructive defects in ventilation. When the defect in ventilation is due to a limitation on chest expansion, the defect is called a *restrictive defect*. Pathologic conditions that limit chest expansion are conditions, such as fibrosis of the lungs, muscle dystrophy, obesity, and abnormal curvature of the spine. Conditions such as pulmonary congestion may cause both obstruction and restriction of ventilation. The ventilation tests help delineate the type of defect present, and whether the defects are reversible with therapy, such as bronchodilators. Ventilation tests are often ordered before a patient has surgery, so any respiratory problems can be anticipated and better treated or prevented.

Pretest Nursing Implications

The clinician conducting the pulmonary function test will give the patient specific instructions for each step of the test. The patient must breathe only through his or her mouth. A noseclip is used on the nose. The patient needs to rest before the test so that he or she can perform as well as possible. The patient should not have any bronchodilators or narcotics before the test because they can change breathing capabilities (Traver, 1974). Because the various breathing maneuvers require the maximal cooperation of the patient, the test is not reliable in young children or confused adults. Food and fluids are not withheld.

Nurses, in ambulatory settings, may be actively involved in actually doing the ventilation tests as one part of a nursing assessment. In one nurse-directed clinic for patients with chronic lung disease, the nurses routinely did FEV, FEV_1 to VC ratios, and MVV (Nield, 1974).

Posttest Nursing Implications

There is no special patient aftercare. The patient may need to rest. He or she may be discouraged if the tests showed less than optimal lung functioning. Poor test results may be an incentive for the patient to stop smoking to prevent further damage. Also, the test results can help guide the nurse in determining what breathing exercises may be beneficial for the patient. Patients with restrictive defects may need help to maximize respiration. Patients with obstructive defects need to learn how to get more air out (pursed lip breathing, etc.). Nurses skilled in teaching breathing techniques use routine spirometry to assess changes in the patient. The clinical significance of some of the basic findings are summarized below.

Summary of Findings from Ventilation Studies

VC and FVC. The vital capacity (VC) is the maximum amount of air that can be expired after a normal inspiration. The forced vital capacity (FVC) is the vital capacity when the breathing is forced.

Reference Values:

Must be determined by charts, which are specific for sex, age, and height. A value less than 80 percent the predicted value would be abnormal.

Clinical Significance. For most patients the results of VC and FVC are similar. Vital capacity increases with physical fitness. In restrictive diseases, the VC or FVC is always decreased—this test is the best assessment of restrictive defects. In obstructive defects, the VC may not be appreciably decreased. However, the more severe the obstruction, the more likely that the air trapping will reduce vital capacity.

FEV. The forced expiratory volume (FEV) is the percentage of vital capacity, which can be expressed in one, two, or three seconds. The figures are expressed as FEV_1, FEV_2, and FEV_3. The test is useful to evaluate the severity of airway obstruction and to evaluate the effectiveness of bronchodilators.

Reference Values:

Normally 65 to 85 percent of the vital capacity can be expressed in the first second and up to 95 and 97 percent by three seconds. For FEV_1, less than 80 percent of the predicted value is considered abnormally low.

Clinical Significance. In obstructive disease, the FEV_1 is decreased. In restrictive disease, the FEV_1 is normal or can be decreased. In some restrictive diseases where there is an increase of elastic resistance, the FEV_1 may be normal or elevated.

Ratio of FEV_1 to FVC.

Reference Values:

Younger people can expell 75 to 85 percent of the VC in one second. Older people can normally expell about 65 to 75 percent in the first second. This is the only pulmonary function test where age is an important determinant and where increases as well as decreases may be abnormal (Boyce and King, 1980).

Clinical Significance. The ratio of the total FVC to FEV_1 is decreased with obstructive disease, and increased, normal, or sometimes decreased with restrictive disease.

VE, MVV, or MBC. These tests measure the volume exhaled in a minute. The volume exhaled per minute at rest is the VE. The volume exhaled in a minute when the person breathes as deeply and rapidly as possible is called the maximum voluntary ventilation (MVV) or the maximal breathing capacity (MBC).

Reference Values:

Values are matched on a chart for age and weight. Less than 80 percent of predicted value is considered abnormally low.

Clinical Significance. Patients with obstructive defects have volumes less than 80 percent of the predicted values. In restrictive disease, the values will usually be normal. Very severe ventilation defects may show less than 35 percent of predicted value.

FEF. This test of forced expiratory flows (FEF) measures how fast a person can exhale a specific amount of air. This test is useful in screening patients for subclinical obstructive disease.

Reference Values:

Values are matched on a chart for age and weight. Less than 75 percent of the predicted value is abnormally low.

Clinical Significance. A long-time smoker may have no symptoms of respiratory problems but the FEF will be less than 75 percent of the predicted values.

In summary, the test used most often for restrictive defects is the FVC. The tests used for obstructive defects are the FEV, FEV_1 to FVC ratio, MVV, and FEF for subclinical cases. For mixed types of defects, all of these tests will be helpful. The programmed instruction by Boyce & King (1980) is excellent for the reader who wishes detailed explanations about the use of the above pulmonary function tests. Fishbach (1980) discusses the less common pulmonary function tests.

THERMOGRAPHY

Description: Thermography is a technique that uses an infrared camera to photograph the surface temperature of the body. The pictures of the temperature of the skin's surface can show variations from cold blue to red hot. The body part to be photographed is exposed to air. The patient is disrobed in a 68 to 70 degree environment for 15 minutes. Some methods involve spraying the area with 95 percent alcohol. Inflammation and malignant processes, where there is an accelerated local metabolism, generate additional heat, which may be detected on the body surface.

Purposes: The most common use for thermography has been as a possible diagnostic tool for cancer of the breast. Different patterns are found in premenopausal and postmenopausal women. For premenopausal women, the breast tissue is more thermally active. At the present time, thermography is not recommended as a screening device for breast cancer because the results are not conclusive (Luckmann & Sorensen, 1980).

Some research has been done to see if thermography can help detect bone tumors, vascular disease, or conditions where inflammation is present. For example, thermography has been suggested as a possible way to measure reactions to skin tests (French, 1980). Thermography is not routinely used clinically at the present time but some studies are being done. For example, thermography is being used to assess areas of pain in the body. The locus of pain is often cooler than the rest of the body (Friedman, 1981). Because thermography is noninvasive, with no risk to the patient, it may be a diagnostic tool that will become more useful in clinical practice in the future.

Questions

1. Special consent forms for noninvasive diagnostic tests are

a. Usually required and are obtained by the physician in charge

b. Always required if the patient has not had the test before

c. Not usually required because there is no risk for the patient
d. Done if the patient is fearful of the procedure

2. The repolarization of the ventricle is shown on the ECG as the

a. QRS complex
b. Q–T interval
c. S–T segment
d. T-wave

3. The characteristics of a normal ECG for an adult include all but

a. A P–R interval less than 0.10 second
b. A heart rate between 60 and 100
c. A positive deflection of the QRS complex on Lead II
d. A P-wave before each QRS complex

4. Premature heart beats change the appearance of the ECG. Which of the following is a characteristic of a premature ventricular contraction?

a. A P-wave precedes the QRS complex
b. A T-wave is absent after the QRS complex
c. The QRS complex is wider than normal
d. The QRS complex is absent

5. Mr. Smiley has just had an ECG done. The nurse has noted that the rhythm seems regular and that there are 8 QRS complexes in 30 large squares of the ECG graph. Therefore, Mr. Smiley's pulse rate is

a. 50
b. 60
c. 70
d. 80

6. Another way to figure Mr. Smiley's pulse rate on the ECG graph would be to count the large squares between each QRS complex. If there were 4 large squares between each QRS complex, Mr. Smiley's rate would be

a. 55
b. 65
c. 75
d. 85

7. Mr. Faber has a history of angina. He had some nonspecific changes on an ECG done today. He is now on telemetry. Which of the following measures of cardiac activity would *not* be necessary by the nurse because telemetry is being used? (Assume the telemetry has been checked and is functioning properly.)

a. Counting the apical rate and noting the rhythm
b. Noting any dyspnea, angina, or abnormal breath sounds
c. Checking the quality of peripheral pulses
d. Noting the amount of urinary output

8. A graphic recording of the force of the cardiac output is called a(n)

a. Vectorcardiogram
b. Phonocardiogram
c. Echocardiogram
d. Ballistogram

9. Which of the following nursing actions is *inappropriate* when the patient is to have an EEG?

a. Allowing a child to nap before the procedure
b. Seeing that the patient has a shampoo
c. Allowing regular meals but no coffee, tea, or colas
d. Checking to see if tranquilizers and sedatives should be withheld

10. Mrs. Tooler is to have an EMG to assess a weakness in her left leg. Which of the following statements is correct to tell Mrs. Tooler when she asks about the test?

a. There is no pain or discomfort during an EMG
b. The test can specifically determine the type of muscular disorder present
c. The patient must remain on bedrest for a while after the test
d. The test can help the physician determine whether the muscular problem is due to nerve or muscle dysfunction

11. Which one of the following pulmonary function tests is most useful for detecting subclinical cases of obstructive defects in ventilation?

a. FVC (Forced vital capacity)
b. FEV_1 (Forced expiratory volume in 1 second)
c. MVV (Maximum voluntary ventilation)
d. FEF (Forced expiratory flow)

12. Pulmonary function tests with a spirometer may be useful in all these clinical situations *except*

a. Mr. Harris, who is going to surgery for an exploratory thoracotomy
b. Mr. Warzyniak, who is a heavy smoker
c. Mr. Leonard, who took an overdose of a narcotic and had respiratory depression for a few hours
d. Sandy Blake, age 15, who has a history of severe asthmatic attacks

13. Thermography is based on the principle that inflammation and some malignant processes cause accelerated heat production. This increase in heat is measured by

a. Rectal and oral thermometers
b. Pictures with an infrared camera
c. Heat-sensitive electrodes attached to the body
d. Immersion in a water bath of a certain temperature

REFERENCES

Allen, B. "Monitoring Cardiovascular Status with Non-Invasive Techniques." *Nursing Clinics of North America* 13: 423–436 (September 1978).

Alspach, J. "Electrical Axis: How to Recognize Deviations on the ECG and Interpret Them." *American Journal of Nursing* 79: 76–83 (November 1979).

Boyce, B. & King, T. "Pulmonary Function Tests in Patient Care." *American Journal of Nursing* 80: 1135–1159 (June 1980).

Bubb, D. "Helping Your Patient Through Two Painful Tests." *RN* 45: 64–65 (January 1982).

Coats, K. "Non-Invasive Cardiac Diagnostic Procedures." *American Journal of Nursing* 75: 1980–1985 (November 1975).

Coats, K. "Techniques in Cardiac Diagnosis." *Nursing Clinics of North America* 11: 259–269 (June 1976).

Corbett, J. *Laboratory Tests In Nursing Practice*. Norwalk, CT: Appleton-Century-Crofts, 1982.

Disch, J. *Diagnostic Procedures for Cardiovascular Disease*. Norwalk, CT: Appleton-Century-Crofts, 1980.

Fishbach, F. *A Manual of Laboratory Tests*. Philadelphia: J. B. Lippincott Company, 1980.

French, R. *Guide to Diagnostic Procedures*. New York: McGraw-Hill, 1980.

Friedman, E. "Imaging Technology Approaches the Frontiers of Physics." *Hospital* 55: 76–78 (January 1981).

Luckmann, J. & Sorensen, K. *Medical-Surgical Nursing: A Psychophysiologic Approach*, 2nd ed. Philadelphia: W. B. Saunders, 1980.

McNeal, G. "Twenty-Four Hour Ambulatory Monitoring." *Nursing Clinics of North America* 13: 437–447 (September 1978).

Meth, I. "Electrical Safety in the Hospital." *American Journal of Nursing* 80: 1344–1348 (July 1980).

Miller, B. & Keane, C. *Encyclopedia and Dictionary of Medicine, Nursing and Allied Health*. Philadelphia: W. B. Saunders, 1978.

Nield, M. A. "A Nurse Directed Chest Clinic." *Nursing Clinics of North America* 9: 147–155 (March 1974).

Pacific Telephone Company. "Heartbeats Sent by Telephone Help Detect Heart Ailments." *Openline* (March 1981).

Phipps, W. et al. *Medical-Surgical Nursing: Concepts and Clinical Practice*, St. Louis: C. V. Mosby Co., 1979.

Price, S. and Wilson, L. *Pathophysiology: Clinical Concepts of Disease Processes*. New York: McGraw-Hill, 1978.

Ross, A. "Neuromuscular Diagnostic Procedures." *Nursing Clinics of North America* 14: 107–121 (March 1979).

Shearer, D. et al. "Preparing a Patient for EEG." *American Journal of Nursing* 77: 63–64 (January 1975).

Spiegel, M. "Electromyoneurography." *American Family Practice* 18: 119–130 (November 1978).

Streiff, L. "Need to Track Your Patient's Heart? Try Telephones and Tape Recorders." *Nursing 81*(11): 74–77 (February 1981).

Taylor, J. & Ballenger, S. *Neurological Dysfunction and Nursing Intervention*. New York: McGraw-Hill, 1980.

Traver, G. "The Nurse's Role in Clinical Testing of Lung Function." *Nursing Clinics of North America* 9: 101–110 (March 1974).

Vaz, D. ''Recognizing Common Cardiac Arrhythmias.'' *American Journal of Nursing* 79: 1971–1975 (November 1979).

Wenger, N. et al. *Cardiology for Nurses*. New York: McGraw-Hill, 1980.

Westfall, U. ''Electrical and Mechanical Events in the Cardiac Cycle.'' *American Journal of Nursing* 76: 231–235 (February 1976).

Wiley, H. & Eaglstein, W. ''Calcinosis Cutis in Children Following Electroencephalography.'' *Journal of the American Medical Association* 242: 455–457 (August 3, 1979).

CHAPTER SIX

Common Invasive Tests

Objectives

1. Identify routine nursing actions in preparing adults and children for invasive diagnostic procedures done at their bedsides, in a treatment room, or outpatient department.
2. Identify the key nursing implications for patients having bone marrow aspirations.
3. Describe the usual procedure for the collection of spinal fluid and the normal characteristics of CSF as demonstrated by routine laboratory analysis.
4. Compare and contrast the pre- and postcare of patients having a thoracentesis or paracentesis.
5. Describe the procedures needed for a gastric analysis, including the use of medications, which may be given by the nurse.
6. Compare and contrast the pre- and postcare of patients having renal and liver biopsies.
7. Identify the key nursing implications for patients having breast and cervical biopsies for potential malignancies.
8. Using the American Cancer Society's recommendations, prepare a teaching project to inform consumers about the Papanicolaou smear as a cancer detection tool.

As discussed in Chapter 5, the division of diagnostic tests into invasive and noninvasive testing is somewhat artificial because all testing may be considered as an invasion of the person to some degree. The term "invasive" is usually used to describe diagnostic tests that entail the use of needles or instruments inserted inside the body to directly record or assess the structure and function of an organ. Some invasive diagnostic procedures are done at the patient's bedside, such as a thoracentesis or pleural tap. Others are done in specially equipped treatment rooms, radiology suites, or even in a very specialized laboratory, such as the cardiac catheterization laboratory. Invasive tests require specialized equipment and highly skilled clinicians. When invasive procedures are done by experienced, skilled clinicians, the incidence of serious side effects is low. But there is always the possibility of complications when the body is invaded by needles and other types of probes. The possibility of complications ranges from minor problems to severe injury and even death. After the physician explains the possible risks to the patient and the expected benefits of the test, the patient or guardian must sign a specific consent form for a particular test. The policy of an informed consent is essential for all invasive tests.

The invasive tests covered in this chapter are those that are usually done in the hospital unit or in an outpatient clinic. A nurse is often present during these procedures and actively assists the physician and supports the patient. These tests include needle aspirations and various kinds of biopsies done under local anesthesia. Nurse practitioners may actually perform selected procedures for stable patients.

The second broad type of invasive procedures are those done in a special laboratory or specially equipped procedure room, such as endoscopic procedures or cardiac catheterizations. The role of the staff nurse for these very specialized procedures is to prepare the patient for the test and to care for the patient afterwards. If a nurse wants to be an assistant with endoscopic procedures or cardiac catheterization, some special clinical training is required. Cardiac catheterizations are discussed in Chapter 7 and endoscopic procedures in Chapter 8.

GENERAL PRETEST NURSING IMPLICATIONS

Collecting Baseline Data

As mentioned earlier, the physician must have the patient or guardian sign a specific consent form for any invasive procedure. The nurse must be aware of the specific policy of the institution. Most institutions also require routine laboratory tests before invasive procedures. The nurse coordinates the collection of any samples needed for laboratory analysis, such as blood coagulation studies (Prothrombin time or PT and Activated Partial Thromboplastin Time APTT), hematocrit (Hct), and urinalysis (UA). The nurse also assesses the physical and mental status of the patient before the test; these are baseline assessments, which are referred to after the test. One of the most critical baseline assessments is the patient's normal blood pressure and pulse rate. For some of these tests, the blood pressure cuff is left on the patient's arm during the procedure so the nurse can take readings throughout the procedure.

Preparing the Patient for Discomfort or Pain

All of the invasive procedures are to some degree uncomfortable for the patient, and most cause a certain amount of pain. At the very least, the pain is confined to the prick accompanying the injection of the local anesthetic. Some procedures also cause momentary pain or unpleasantness during the test. If the nurse is with the patient during the procedure, he or she can be very valuable in assisting the patient to deal with any expected momentary pain. For example, various breathing techniques or pain distractors can be taught to the patient. Sometimes just squeezing the nurse's hand will help the patient cope. Depending on the interest of the patient and the skill of the nurse, the patient may be taught techniques, such as imaging or other ways, to divert his or her attention from the present situation. For example, if the patient has learned the LaMaze breathing technique to reduce discomfort during labor, this technique could be used to lessen the discomfort during a painful procedure. The nurse should find out what the patient thinks will be a help to ease discomfort. For some patients sedatives may be needed, but accurate information about the test may alleviate anxiety and make sedatives unnecessary. The key points to emphasize are that 1) the duration of pain will be very brief and, 2) local anesthetics will be used. Pretest information should include what the person will see, smell, taste, or feel to lessen the dread of the unknown. Some patients may want a lot of technical information. Others may want to know *only* how much it will hurt. Research studies have demonstrated that adult patients who receive information about the "sensations" of a procedure appear to have less anxiety than patients who receive no information or only procedural information (Johnson, 1978).

Special Needs of Children

Preparing children for invasive tests means preparing the parents, too. It is sometimes better to let the parents do the explaining to the child. It has been suggested that it is better to tell the adolescent when he or she is alone (Pidgeon, 1977). The nurse's assessment of the child's growth and developmental stage is essential for appropriate health teaching. Encouraging a young child to play with some of the equipment may help alleviate anxiety. Research studies have suggested that, as with adults, telling the child about the "sensations" he will feel may lower distress (Johnson et al., 1975). Adolescents may be particularly interested in seeing what equipment will be used during the test. Children, as well as adults, need to know how they can help during the test. Young children may have to be restrained; thus, they deserve explanations. By age three, it may be possible to do procedures without the use of a restraint if 1) the parent holds the child, 2) the child is allowed to participate, and 3) acceptable behavior is rewarded (Beckemeyer & Bahr, 1980). Keeping a security blanket or favorite toy nearby may also help relieve the child's anxiety.

Explanation of Aftercare Procedures

The nurse also needs to explain what aftercare will be needed. Thus, children and parents will not be concerned because the child is being carefully watched after the test. By the same token, the adolescent or adult needs to be told before the test that his or her blood pressure will be taken, say, every fifteen minutes so there is no misconception that something is amiss.

Use of Special Trays

For all of these procedures, special trays are used. For example, the basic equipment for a lumbar puncture (L.P.) is sterilized on one tray. A check must be done to see if the necessary slides, chemistry tubes, culture tubes, etc. are included on a special procedure tray. Someone may need to check with the laboratory to determine what tubes are necessary to collect.

In some institutions, the nurse may be responsible for setting up equipment for a procedure. In other settings, the person who performs the procedure is responsible for acquiring all needed equipment. Many procedure trays are now packaged commercially with all disposable items. The nurse must check with the particular institutions to see exactly what procedures are followed in that setting.

Use of Antiseptic Solutions

Most prepared trays contain packets of skin antiseptics, such as povidone-iodine (Betadine), which has broad spectrum microbicidal action.

Equipment for Local Anesthesia

The syringes and needles used for the local anesthetic are included on the various trays. Three routine types of needles on a procedure tray are: 1) 25-gauge ⅝-inch needles for local skin infiltration, 2) 22-gauge 1½-inch needles for deeper structures, and 3) spinal needles, which are various gauges and extra long (over three inches) for very deep injections. (Note that specific trays, such as a bone marrow or paracentesis tray, will also include specific cutting needles or trocars for different test procedures.) Sterile towels are also on prepared procedure trays. Usually the vial of anesthetic is not included on the equipment tray and must be added.

Types of Local Anesthetics

The two most common local anesthetics used for invasive diagnostic testing are procaine (Novocaine) and lidocaine (Xylocaine). Procaine lasts about ¾ to 1½ hours; lidocaine lasts for 1½ to 2 hours. Sometimes a very small amount of epinephrine (adrenalin) is combined with a local anesthetic agent to promote local vasoconstriction. Two reasons why some local vasoconstriction may be desirable are: 1) the vasoconstriction slows down the absorption of the drug to lengthen its duration and 2) the vasoconstriction may cause decreased bleeding at the injection site. Note that epinephrine is not used in areas of the body supplied by end-arteries; such as "fingers, toes, penis, or nose." Epinephrine is never used with a local anesthetic if tissue circulation is compromised.

Adverse Reactions to Local Anesthetics

Systemic effects can arise from local injections containing epinephrine. Nurses should assess for any skin flush or increased pulse when epinephrine is used. Anaphylaxis can occur from lidocaine or procaine if the patient is allergic to local anesthetics. Nurses must assess for allergies before any drugs are given. Emergency drugs and equipment for resuscitation should always be available when an invasive test is performed. Preparation for the unexpected is as important in an outpatient setting as in a hospital setting.

Arranging Environment for the Test

The nurse or clinician doing the procedure must check the lighting in the area. Most hospitals have a treatment room, which ensures adequate lighting and privacy. If the procedure is done at the patient's bedside, a treatment light should be brought to the room. A good light is needed so doors do not have to be open—closed doors ensure privacy for the patient. In a multiple bed unit, it is better to take the patient to a treatment room, otherwise, the bed should be screened and perhaps the other patient can go to a waiting room, if possible. Patients should not be exposed to another patient's invasive procedure.

Physical Preparation of the Patient

Some of the tests require the patient to maintain n.p.o. status, while others do not. Medications may or may not be withheld; specific medications may be part of the test. The patient should be physically comfortable; thus, he or she should be given a chance to void before the procedure begins. (For some of the procedures, such as a paracentesis, an empty bladder is essential.) The specific physical preparation for the patient is covered under the discussion for each individual test. (See Table 9 for key points about the tests.)

Nurse's Role During Procedure

The nurse may remain with the patient to offer support. It has already been stressed that the nurse can help prepare the patient for the procedure by exploring, with the patient, the best way to cope with any pain or discomfort. The nurse can explain that the antiseptic will feel cold to the skin and the injection of the local anesthetic will cause a stinging sensation. The nurse can offer to hold the patient's hand or let the patient squeeze his or her hand. Hand holding also helps remind the patient not to put his or her hands on the sterile field. For a child, special restraining procedures may be required to ensure the safety of the child and the sterility of the procedure. The parent may help hold the child. If the parent is not present, the nurse can hold the child. The nurse may be essential in helping the patient maintain a certain position, such as with a lumbar puncture. The nurse also assists the physician or the clinician, who is actually doing the procedure. This may require pouring an antiseptic into a basin, opening extra gauze packages, holding collection tubes, etc. The nurse must make sure all collected samples are clearly marked in the order collected. Also, the nurse is needed to observe any untoward effects of the procedure, e.g., check the blood pressure several times during a procedure.

With the expanding role of the nurse, a nurse-practitioner may actually perform the test (Markus, 1981). Nurse-practitioners do bone marrow aspirations on patients as part of their caseloads. However, the focus of this chapter is for the nurse in general practice, who is, usually the assistant during invasive diagnostic procedures. Cosgriff (1978) gives detailed steps and pictures of the common diagnostic procedures, with special tips for the clinician during the procedure.

GENERAL POSTTEST NURSING IMPLICATIONS

Checking Vital Signs

One of the nursing implications for any invasive test is to carefully check vital signs before, during, and after the procedure. Typical orders after an invasive procedure would be vital signs every 15 minutes for one hour, then every hour for four hours, and then routine if stable (Tucker, 1980). Routines may vary for different procedures, depending on the policy of the specific institution and the exact procedure done. The nurse should take the VS more often if there is any apparent unstability. Regardless of the stability of the vital signs, they should be taken at regular intervals as long as there is any possibility of the patient bleeding or having other complications. Vitals signs after an invasive test include blood pressure, pulse, and respiration. The patient's temperature is *not* taken every 15 minutes. The patient's temperature may become more important later if there is any possibility that the procedure caused an infection. If there is any indication of possible

TABLE 9. COMMON INVASIVE TESTS: SUMMARY OF KEY POINTS FOR NURSING CARE[a]

Test	N.P.O. Status Pretest?	Local Anesthetic Used?	Restricted Activity Posttest?	Assess for Complications?
Lumbar puncture	Varies	Yes	Varies, usually several hours	Spinal headache; nerve damage to legs or bladder
Bone marrow biopsy	No	Yes	No	None likely; infection possible
Thoracentesis	No	Yes	1 hour on affected side	Pneumothorax; subcutaneous emphysema
Paracentesis	No	Yes	No	Hypovolemia; peritonitis
Gastric analysis	Yes	No	No	Possible allergic reaction to histamine-type drugs
Papanicolaou smears of uterus	No	No	No	None likely
Cervical biopsy	No	No	No	Bleeding from biopsy site
Breast biopsy	No	Yes	No	None likely; infection at site or bleeding possible
Liver biopsy	Yes	Yes	Up to 24 hours	Internal bleeding; bile peritonitis
Renal biopsy	No	Yes	Up to 24 hours	Hematuria and internal bleeding; urinary tract infection

[a] *See text for more detailed discussions about all preparations before and after each test.*

febrile reactions, then temperature should be checked routinely every four hours. All vital signs must be documented on the patient's record and should be graphed so trends (i.e., decreasing blood pressure and increasing pulse rate) are readily apparent.

Charting

The time and the name of the clinician, who performed the procedure, should be recorded. The amount of any fluid withdrawn and its color and characteristics (i.e., cloudy or bloody) should be noted. The number of specimens sent to the laboratory should also be documented.

In addition to the specific items, such as the vital signs and other items discussed later, the nurse should record the general condition of the patient after the test. For example, if there were no untoward reactions, this should be noted as "patient tolerated procedure well with no complications noted at present." *Specific* assessments for the patient's condition depend on the test. These are emphasized in the discussion about each test.

Positioning and Bedrest

The positioning of the patient after the procedure may be important. If the patient is to remain in a certain position or on bedrest for a specified amount of time, the patient needs to know this information. Also a sign can be placed at the foot of the bed. For example, the sign may say "Keep flat in bed until 7 P.M." Information about positioning should also be recorded in the Kardex.

Assessing for Pain and Complications

The nurse must know what type of pain is usual after a procedure so ordered analgesics can be used for relief without masking what could be a symptom of a complication. The nurse must also know any specific complications associated with a procedure so the posttest assessment is appropriate. For example, listening for breath sounds after a pleural tap or thoracentesis is necessary to detect a pneumothorax. There may be follow-up laboratory work, such as hematocrits to assess for blood loss.

Changing Dressings

The dressing over the site of an invasive procedure should remain sterile. The nurse must use sterile technique if the dressing becomes wet and needs to be changed. Some procedures may require a pressure dressing with a sandbag, while others only require a small adhesive dressing.

Resuming Oral Intake

Any limitations on eating after the procedure will be discussed for the specific tests. For some tests, encouraging fluids is beneficial.

LUMBAR PUNCTURE

Description: Positioning of the patient for a lumbar puncture (L.P.) is very important. Patients are turned on their sides and told to curl up into a ball with head and feet as close to each other as possible (fetal position). This position allows for the maximum separation of the vertebrae. A lumbar puncture can be done with the patient in a sitting position, but pressure readings cannot be obtained. The usual preparation of the skin with antiseptic and local anesthetic is done. The clinician inserts a spinal needle into a lumbar space, which is below the end of the spinal cord. The spinal cord usually terminates at the second lumbar vertebra. Thus, the spinal cord is not touched by the needle. Sometimes the needle does glaze a spinal root causing a sharp pain, which radiates down the patient's leg (Taylor & Ballenger, 1980). If the patient has pain in one of the legs, the clinician needs to know which leg, so the needle position can be slightly readjusted. Once the needle is positioned in the sub-arachnoid space, a pressure reading is taken with a three-way stopcock and a manometer (standard equipment on an L.P. tray). The patient must relax and straighten out his or her legs before the opening pressure is done because intraabdominal pressure will increase cerebrospinal fluid (CSF) pressure. After a baseline pressure has been obtained, the physician may want the patient to strain slightly (Valsalva's maneuver) to see if the increased abdominal pressure causes an increase in CSF pressure. If there is a blockage in the spinal canal, the CSF pressure may not change. The Queckenstedt test is also used to see if there is a block in the flow of CSF. The physician may ask the nurse to apply finger pressure to both internal jugular veins of the patient. Obstruction of these veins will cause a rise in CSF pressure, unless there is a block somewhere in the spinal column. The Queckenstedt test can be dangerous if too much pressure is put on the carotid receptors. The assistant must know exactly how and where to apply the pressure. After the pressure readings are done, a few milliliters of CSF are obtained in tubes for 1) chemistry, 2) cell counts, and 3) microbiology. A closing pressure may be obtained. The CSF pressure drops 5 to 10 mm of water pressure for each milliliter of fluid removed. Usually only about 10 ml are removed, but this can reduce pressure by 50 to 100 mm (Cosgriff, 1978). The needle is withdrawn and a dry sterile dressing is placed over the site.

Purposes: A lumbar puncture or spinal tap measures cerebral spinal fluid pressure and is used to obtain cerebral spinal fluid for laboratory examination. A lumbar puncture is also done to inject dye into the spinal column (see myelograms, Chapter 1). The lumbar puncture done for a spinal tap is similar in type of procedure to that done for spinal anesthetics.

Spinal fluid is formed in the lateral ventricles in the brain. The fluid bathes the brain and spinal cord and protects the central nervous system from injury. Measurements of the various cerebrospinal fluid components helps in the diagnosis of various conditions of the central nervous system. A special summary about the clinical significance of CSF changes is covered at the end of this section. Nurses should be aware of the normal characteristics of CSF because the laboratory results are usually sent to the unit.

Contraindications for L.P.

A measurement of the CSF pressure will help detect any obstruction in the normal flow of the CSF. However, if increased intracranial pressure is suspected, a lumbar puncture is *not* attempted because a quick reduction in the pressure in the spinal column can cause a herniation of the brain stem into the foramen magnum. This downward shift of the brain can put lethal pressure on the vital centers in the medulla.

Pretest Nursing Implications

Note the general implications for all invasive testing, e.g., policy on consent forms. The patient does not need to maintain n.p.o. status for an L.P. Sedation is usually not used, but may be necessary for children or confused adults. A blood glucose sample must be drawn about a half hour to an hour before the test to be used as a comparison for the CSF glucose level. A serum chloride level may be used for comparison too, but this is not routine.

Posttest Nursing Implications

Assessing for Change in Neuro Functioning. See the general guidelines about vital signs, assessing for pain, etc. Special attention should be paid to any change in the level of consciousness, particularly if increased intracranial pressure is suspected. The patient may have a temporary problem in voiding due to the effect on nerves to the bladder.

Positioning of Patient. Positioning of the patient after an L.P. may or may not be a critical issue. More commonly, the patient may be instructed to stay flat in bed for several hours to prevent any spinal headaches. If the lumbar puncture is done on an outpatient basis, the patient may be allowed to go home without being prone for a period (Phipps et al., 1979).

Assessing and Intervening for Spinal Headaches. The exact reason for a spinal headache is not known, but it is assumed to be related to the loss of cerebral spinal fluid. The use of a large needle (18-gauge) or other trauma during the procedure may cause more loss of spinal fluid, and thus, there is less fluid to bathe the meninges of the brain. Petito and Plum (1974) advocate that a patient lie prone for only three hours after an L.P. because they believe it is the size of the needle that causes the headache, more than the position afterwards. If a headache does begin, the patient is maintained on bedrest with an icecap and mild analgesics given as ordered. The spinal headache usually goes away in 24 hours, but it may persist longer, sometimes for weeks.

Encouraging Fluids. After an L.P., the patient can eat and drink as soon as he or she desires. Unless otherwise contraindicated, drinking plenty of fluids should be encouraged because this helps the body replace any lost CSF.

Reference Values (Sculley, 1980)

- Bilirubin: negative.
- Cell count: 0–5 cell lymphocytes/mL—infants and young children up to 20, some may be polymorphonuclears, not just lymphs.
- Chloride: 120–130 mEq/liter—compare with serum, should be 10 mEq higher
- Glucose: 50–75 mg/dl—compare with serum glucose, should be 20 mg less.
- Protein: 15–45 mg/dl
  Albumin: 21 mg/dl
  IgG: 3.4 mg/dl.
- Pressure: 70–180 mmH_2O—infants and young children, 50–100 mmH_2O.

General Significance of Abnormal Findings in CSF

Blood in the Fluid. Normally, the fluid should be very clear in color. Bleeding from the tap itself will usually not make all the tubes bloody. The collection of samples should be marked as #1, #2, and #3 so it is possible to see if the blood is less in the last tube than in the first tube. If the CSF is grossly bloody, this is a sign of hemorrhage somewhere in the central nervous system. It may not be possible to do any other tests on the CSF when a great deal of blood is present.

Bilirubin. Bilirubin (the indirect portion) can cross the blood brain barrier in infants. (Note that bilirubin in the spinal fluid of the newborn (Kernicterus) can cause brain damage.)

Cell Counts. Normally there are fewer than five cells per mL in CSF, all are lymphocytes. In bacterial infections there may be enough neutrophils to make the CSF cloudy. In tuberculosis and some viral diseases lymphocytes may be increased. Tumor cells can also be identified by a Papanicolaou smear.

Chlorides. Chlorides are decreased in some bacterial infections, including tuberculosis. This test is not specific enough to be of much use and is not done anymore unless specifically requested (Koepke, 1980).

Glucose. The glucose level is lowered in bacterial infections because the bacteria utilize sugar. Some types of tumors may also cause a lowered CSF sugar. The blood glucose sample is needed for a comparison. Ideally the blood glucose sample is drawn about 30 minutes before the L.P. because it takes glucose about 30 minutes to an hour to diffuse into the CSF.

Proteins. Degenerative diseases and brain tumors tend to cause increased protein in the CSF. Structural lesions that interrupt the blood brain barrier cause increased total protein in the CSF because there is increased diffusion from the blood to the brain tissue. In general, an increase in the total protein of the CSF is a sign of a serious neurologic disorder, but the total protein is not specifically diagnostic. Because various diseases cause elevations in only certain types of proteins, much research is directed toward identifying exactly what types of proteins are elevated in various diseases of the central nervous system. For example, demyelinating diseases of the central nervous system are those in which the myelin sheath covering the neurons is lost (Taylor & Ballenger, 1980). During active demyelination a basic protein is present in the serum, as well as the CSF. Basic protein tests may someday be used to identify such diseases as multiple sclerosis, a demyelinating disease (Cohen et al., 1976). Immunoelectrophoresis can be done on CSF, as well as on serum and urine, to identify abnormal proteins.

Gram Stains and Cultures

Cultures are done to identify any organisms found in the CSF. If a preliminary gram stain identifies any organisms, the physician is notified immediately so treatment can begin at once.

Serologic Tests

The laboratory may do various types of serologic tests to determine the presence of neurosyphilis. See Corbett (1982) for examples of serologic tests for syphilis (STS).

BONE MARROW ASPIRATION OR BONE MARROW BIOPSY

Description: Common sites used for the adult in order of preference are posterior iliac crest, anterior iliac crest, and sternum. The tibia may be used in a small child (Barber et al., 1977). If a biopsy, rather than just an aspiration, is planned, the iliac crest is used. The area is prepped and a local anesthetic is used. Hair may have to be shaved from the site. The physician or nurse-practitioner inserts the needle through the bone until the marrow is reached. For an aspiration, the plunger of the syringe is pulled back to withdraw a little bit of the marrow into the syringe. When the plunger is pulled back, the patient often feels sharp pain. The patient should be prepared for this momentary pain. Normal bone marrow is soft and semifluid, and thus, a sample can often be obtained by aspiration with a syringe. Otherwise, a bone marrow biopsy can be done with a large-size needle, which has a cutting blade. The specimen obtained must be carefully placed in the correct container. A smear may be microscopically examined immediately to make sure tiny bone particles, called spicules, are present (Markus, 1981). Six or more slides may be done. A culture tube may also be necessary. Usually only a Band-Aid or small adhesive dressing is placed over the site because there is minimal bleeding or drainage. A small pressure dressing is used if a biopsy was done.
Purposes: Bone marrow studies are done when there are abnormal types of cells on a peripheral blood smear. They are used to confirm the presence of metastatic tumors or diseases such as leukemia or various types of anemias. Bone marrow studies may be done periodically to evaluate the response to treatment.

Pretest Nursing Implications

The patient is usually not given sedation, but if sedation is deemed necessary, it does not interfere with the test. The patient can eat and drink before the test. The procedure, including the momentary pain, should be explained to the patient. The patient is positioned with pillows under the thoracic spine if the sternum is used. The iliac crest is done with the patient in a side-lying position or on his or her abdomen. The nurse needs to help the patient get into as comfortable position as possible, so the patient can remain still during the procedure.

Posttest Nursing Implications

Vital signs and other routines are done as for other invasive tests. The patient may stay in bed for an hour or so to rest, but can then resume normal daily activities. Any unusual drainage or bleeding should be reported at once. There may be a slight aching or pain, which requires the use of a mild analgesic.

THORACENTESIS

Description: The site usually used for a thoracentesis (pleural tap) is the seventh or eighth intercostal space (Cosgriff, 1978). The clinician determines the exact site to put the needle by studying the patient's chest x-ray and by percussion and auscultation of the chest. The patient is usually in a sitting position so fluid will pool in the base of the pleural space. If the patient cannot sit up, he or she may be turned toward the unaffected side and placed in a high Fowler's position. The area is prepped and anesthesized. After the needle is positioned in the pleural space, fluid is withdrawn with a syringe and a three-way stopcock. (If the tap is therapeutic, up to 1000 ml may be withdrawn.) The patient may feel some pain as the pleural space is entered, but the withdrawing of fluid is not uncomfortable. Once the fluid is withdrawn, a small bandage is placed over the site. Some clinicians may spray the site with a collodian seal.

Purposes: A thoracentesis is an insertion of a needle into the pleural space with aspiration of air, pleural fluid or blood from the pleural cavity. A thoracentesis is often done for therapy as well as for diagnosis. Inflammatory diseases of the lungs and neoplasms are common reasons for a large collection of pleural fluid. Blood in the pleural space (hemothorax) is usually from a traumatic injury. The thoracentesis is usually done at the patient's bedside or in the procedure room on the unit. Thoracentesis can also be done in an office or clinic setting.

Laboratory Examination of Pleural Fluid

The fluid collected for the laboratory may include 1) chemistry, 2) bacteria, and 3) histopathology. Tumor cells can be identified as well as various organisms.

Pretest Nursing Implications

The general pretest nursing implications for bedside exams are followed. An extra bedside table may be necessary to help position the patient in a comfortable sitting position. The patient can lean over the table with his or her feet on a chair for support. Chest x-rays are needed. The nurse should listen to the patient's breath sounds to be used as a baseline for a posttest assessment. The nurse should also note any breathing difficulty and the color of the patient's skin before the test is begun. Sedation, although not usually used, will not interfere with the procedure if needed. Food, fluids, and medicines do not need to be withheld.

Posttest Nursing Implications

Positioning and Other Routine Care. The patient is usually turned on the *unaffected* side for one hour to allow the pleural puncture to seal. Vital signs are recorded per hospital routine. The amount of fluid withdrawn for diagnosis, if more than a few milliliters, should be recorded as part of the intake and output record. There is no restriction on food or fluids following the procedure. If the patient has no respiratory or other problems within an hour after the test, all normal activity can be resumed. The nurse must check for any signs of hypovolemia. Also, electrolytes may be ordered to evaluate electrolyte balance. Careful note should be made of the respiratory rate and the character of the respirations.

Assessments for Possible Complications. The nurse should listen for any diminished breath sounds, which could be a sign of a pneumothorax. Any dyspnea or shortness of breath should be carefully compared to the respiratory status before the test. If a large amount of fluid was withdrawn as therapy, the patient should be able to breathe with less effort. A chest x-ray is done to evaluate the amount of fluid that was removed and to check for any pneumothorax.

Subcutaneous emphysema is leakage of air into the subcutaneous tissues. The tissues feel like rolled up tissue paper and crackle when touched (crepitus). The air in the tissues is from a leak in the pleural cavity. If the patient has no respiratory problems associated with the crepitus, this air will gradually be reabsorbed without treatment.

Patients with pleural effusion due to malignancies may have cytoxic or antibiotic drugs injected into the pleural space after the fluid is withdrawn. The nurse must be aware of possible reactions to the particular drug injected into the pleural space (Luckmann & Sorensen, 1980).

ABDOMINAL PARACENTESIS

Description: The word *paracentesis* actually means puncture of any cavity for the aspiration of fluid (Miller & Keane, 1978). An abdominal paracentesis is used for the removal of fluid from a peritoneal cavity. In general practice, the abdominal paracentesis is usually just called a paracentesis because withdrawals of fluids from other cavities have specific names (i.e., thoracentesis, aminocentesis, etc.)

A paracentesis is done at the patient's bedside or in an outpatient setting. The patient must sit up with the feet supported. A bedside table may be used to support the arms in a comfortable position. The physician inserts a large-gauge needle or trocar through the abdominal wall. (It is essential that the bladder be empty so there is no accidental puncture of the bladder.) Once the needle is in the peritoneal cavity, the fluid is withdrawn by a syringe if just a small amount is needed for diagnosis. If the tap is also needed to relieve pressure from ascites, the needle may be connected to a tubing and a large collection bottle is used, which is much like the set-up used to withdraw blood. Up to 1000 ml may be withdrawn at one time. A newer technique is to do a slow continuous drainage of ascites. It is possible to take out as much as nine liters in eight hours (Fisher, 1979). The major concern when a large amount of fluid is removed is there may be a shift of fluid from the vascular space to the now-empty peritoneal cavity. Intravenous fluid or albumin may be used to prevent hypotension when large amounts of fluid are withdrawn. Once the needle or trocar is withdrawn, a small sterile dressing is placed over the site. If the patient has a great deal of ascites, and only a small amount of fluid was removed, the pressure of the remaining fluid may cause a continued leakage from the puncture site. The dressing may need to be changed frequently and extra fluff gauze used to absorb the leakage. The use of Montgomery straps eliminates the need to change the tape every time the dressing is changed.

Purposes: A paracentesis may be done to assess for peritonitis. If the patient has had peritoneal dialysis, the specimen may be aspirated from the peritoneal catheter. The nurse may collect this specimen by withdrawing a small amount of fluid via a syringe (Shetler & Bantos, 1981), using sterile technique.

An abnormal collection of fluid in the peritoneal cavity is called *ascites*. Ascites is most often seen in patients with advanced cirrhosis or widespread abdominal malignancies. For these conditions, a paracentesis is done for therapeutic rather than diagnostic reasons. The major drawback of doing a paracentesis for therapeutic reasons is that ascitic fluid contains a significant amount of protein. Because paracentesis causes a loss of protein, other measures, such as diuretics, are used before a paracentesis is done for therapy.

In addition to diagnostic aids or therapeutic relief in cirrhosis and malignancies, paracentesis is also done as a diagnostic procedure for traumatic injuries to the abdomen. A peritoneal tap, or a peritoneal lavage with Ringer's lactate solution, is done to see if there is any bleeding into the peritoneal cavity (Cosgriff, 1978).

Laboratory Examinations of Peritoneal Fluid

Laboratory examination of the peritoneal fluid may include RBC, WBC, cultures, fecal content, bilirubin, and amylase (if pancreatitis is suspected). Normally peritoneal fluid is clear and yellowish. If there is any blood in the fluid, this is abnormal. If the blood is intraperitoneal blood, it will not clot, but if it is venous blood (which was accidentally withdrawn from a vessel), the blood will clot (Cosgriff, 1978). The amount of protein in the fluid helps distinguish a transudate from an exudate. Exudates, which usually result from inflammation, contain more protein than transudates, which are usually due to pressure changes from mechanical factors.

Pretest Nursing Implications

In addition to the general implications for invasive testing, the patient should be weighed before and after the procedure to assess the fluid loss. (Recall that one liter of fluid weighs one kilogram or 2.2 pounds.) The patient *must have* an empty bladder so it is not pricked by the needle. If the patient cannot void, a catheter may be necessary. The patient needs to be in a comfortable sitting position with the feet supported on a bedside stool or chair. When a large amount of fluid is being withdrawn, the patient's blood pressure needs to be taken several times during the procedure. Intravenous equipment should be readily available in case of hypotension from shifts of fluid out of the vascular space. Intravenous albumin is sometimes given immediately after the procedure.

Posttest Nursing Implications

Assessing Fluid and Electrolyte Balance. Vital signs are checked and other routine aftercare for invasive procedures are done. The patient's pre- and postweight should be compared. The exact amount, color, and character of the removed fluid should be noted on the nurse's notes and as part of the intake and output record. The patient should be on I and Q for a period of 24 hours. Depending on the reasons for the ascites, the patient may be on a restricted fluid or sodium diet. Electrolytes must be closely monitored.

Assessing for Other Complications. As noted above, if any excess fluid was left in the peritoneal cavity, there may be a problem with leakage from the site. The dressing may need to be changed frequently. Sterile techniques must be used. The patient's temperature should be taken every four hours for 24 hours. The nurse should carefully observe the patient for other signs or symptoms of a developing peritonitis, such as abdominal pain and tense, rigid abdominal muscles.

GASTRIC ANALYSIS

Description:

Insertion of a Nasogastric Tube. A gastric analysis is usually done at the patient's bedside, in a treatment room, or in an office or clinic. The nurse or physician may insert the tube, which should be well lubricated with a water soluble jelly. The patient is seated in an upright position. The nasogastric tube is passed into the stomach and left for the duration of the test. Either nostril may be used. The patient may know that one side of his nose is more patent than the other side. The patient's head should be hyperextended for the passage of the tube to the back of the throat. Once the tube reaches the posterior pharynx, the patient can put his or her head back in a normal position or slightly forward. Sips of water, unless contraindicated, are given to help the tube go down the esophagus. A slight pulling back on the tube and a slight downward thrust are needed when the tube is felt to touch the posterior pharynx. Passing of a nasogastric tube is an unpleasant experience for the patient. It may be necessary to stop for a moment to let the patient relax. Once the tube is going down the esophagus easily, it should be passed rapidly so that the patient does not gag. (It is possible to stimulate a vagal response by gagging and this can cause bradycardia, which can be dangerous to some patients.) If the nasogastric tube is inadvertently put into the trachea of an alert patient, this mistake will be very obvious because the patient will cough violently and will very actively resist the tube, which is suddenly blocking the air passage. Once the tube is in the stomach, a fasting specimen is obtained by aspiration with a large syringe. Obtaining gastric contents is the best evidence the tube is indeed in the stomach.

Use of Drugs in Gastric Analysis. A drug is given subcutaneously to stimulate gastric secretions, either histamine or a histamine analogue, betazole hydrochloride (Histalog). The patient should be observed for an increased pulse rate and a decreased blood pressure because of the vasodilating properties of histamine and histaminelike drugs. Some patients may experience a warm, flushed feeling or more severe symptoms of an allergic response. Antihistamine drugs and epinephrine should be readily available in the event that the patient does have a severe allergic reaction to the drug. After the drug has been given to stimulate gastric secretions, gastric secretions are taken at certain time intervals. The time of each specimen is marked on each collection tube, and all of the specimens are sent to the laboratory for acidity analysis.

Reference Values (Sculley, 1980)

Basal
- Females: 2.0 ± 1.8 mEq/h
- Males: 3.0 ± 2.0 mEq/h

Maximal (after histalog or gastrin)
- Females: 16 ± 5 mEq/h
- Males: 23 ± 5 mEq/h

Purposes: A gastric analysis is most commonly done to measure the acidity of the gastric contents. The response of the gastric glands to drug stimulation with histamine or histaminelike drugs is helpful in diagnosing a peptic ulcer, gastric carcinoma, and pernicious anemia. Gastric acidity is usually increased with a peptic ulcer and decreased or totally absent (anacidity or achlorhydria) in pernicious anemia and gastric carcinoma. An analysis of gastric contents may also be done to detect acid fast bacillus in the patient with undiagnosed tuberculosis. The patient with tuberculosis usually swallows some sputum containing the organism that causes tuberculosis, which is acid-fast so it is not destroyed by the gastric juices. The gastric contents can also be examined for the presence of malignant cells by doing a Papanicolaou smear. Test for occult blood may also be done.

Insulin may be given to test the stomach's response to vagal stimulation. The vagus nerve causes increased production of hydrochloric acid by the stomach. Hypoglycemia, caused by the insulin, is a stimulus to the vagus. The response of the stomach may be used to evaluate the effect of a vagotomy or to diagnose other problems of gastric acidity. The use of insulin with a gastric analysis is called the Hollander's test (Luckmann & Sorensen, 1980).

Pretest Nursing Implications

It is important that the patient be checked for any history of allergic reactions. If the patient is known to be highly allergic, a small test dose of Histalogue may be given before the test. The patient must maintain n.p.o. status for six to eight hours before the test. The patient should not smoke because it increases the secretion of gastric acid. Also, the patient should not receive anticholinergic drugs, such as atropine, because they markedly decrease gastric secretions by blocking the action of the vagus nerve.

Posttest Nursing Implications

Removing the Nasogastric Tube. Once all specimens are obtained, the nasogastric tube can be removed. The patient should be told that the tube will be removed quickly. The nurse can remove the tube by pinching it and quickly pulling it out. Paper towels should be handy to catch the tube, and the patient will need tissues to blow his or her nose. The patient may want to close his or her eyes or concentrate on something else while the tube is pulled out.

Returning to Normal Activities. There are no restrictions on activity after a gastric analysis. Vital signs are only necessary once or twice to ensure the continued stable condition of the patient. The patient can eat as soon as he or she wishes. A sip of water or some weak, warm tea may be offered first as the patient may prefer to rest for a while.

Tubeless Gastric Analysis. A tubeless gastric analysis uses only tablets to screen for patients who might have gastric hypoacidity. The patient swallows tablets that contain a dye (Diagnex Blue), which is released if hydrochloric acid is present in the stomach. The dye is absorbed and excreted in the urine in a couple of hours. A lack of gastric acidity would be reflected by a lack of dye in the urine. This test is not considered precise enough to be valuable in actually diagnosing hypoacidity. (Insurance carriers, such as Blue Cross, will no longer pay for the test.) Older nursing textbooks sometimes include information on this test.

PAPANICOLAOU SMEARS OR EXFOLIATIVE CYTOLOGIC STUDIES

The Papanicolaou smear usually refers to a test for malignant cells from the uterus, but they can be done of many body secretions. The Papanicolaou smear was named after Dr. George Papanicolaou who, in the 1940s, developed a technique for identifying malignant cells in body secretions. Malignant cells slough off (exfoliate) more readily than do normal cells. The field that involves Papanicolaou smears is sometimes called *Exfoliative Cytology*. In addition to uteral or cervical secretions, exfoliative cytology studies are done on sputum, pleural fluid, bronchial washings from a bronchoscope, gastric contents, bladder secretions, peritoneal fluid, and even secretions from the mammary glands. The collection of a sample for exfoliative cytology is often part of an invasive study. The laboratory will tell the nurse exactly how the specimen should be prepared. The results of a Papanicolaou smear are reported as:

- Grade I: Normal appearing cells.
- Grade II: Atypical cytology, but no evidence of malignancy.
- Grade III: Suggestion of malignancy, but not conclusive.
- Grade IV: Strongly suggestive of malignancy.
- Grade V: Conclusive of malignancy.

It must be remembered that all reports of exfoliative cytology are used for screening, not for a final diagnosis. Thus, the presence of a malignancy is always confirmed with a biopsy (Phipps et al., 1979).

PAPANICOLAOU SMEARS OF THE UTERUS

Description: A small amount of secretion is obtained from the cervix by swabbing the exterior of the cervix with an applicator. A Gravlee jet washer may be used to get cells from the endometrium. Most sources suggest that two smears should be taken in order to increase the chance of obtaining any atypical cells, which may be present (Rank et al., 1977). The smears are put on dry slides and immediately sprayed with a commercial fixative. It is important that the cells not dry up before they are fixed on the slide.
Purposes: The American Cancer Society used to recommend annual Papanicolaou smears for all women over age 20 or for those under age 20, who were sexually active. The latest recommendation of the American Cancer Society (1980) is that a Papanicolaou smear be done at least every three years, after two initial smears done a year apart are negative. This applies to all women age 20 to 40, as well as sexually active women under age 20. All women over age 40 should continue to have yearly pelvic exams to screen for pelvic cancer. The American College of Obstetricians and Gynecologists (1980) has taken the stand that *yearly* examination of a Papanicolaou smear be done on all adult women regardless of age. They cite that the annual smear is not only useful for detecting cancer but also other problems, which can be detected by a yearly visit to a gynecologist.

Pretest Nursing Implications

The Papanicolaou smear is usually done five to six days after the menses. The patient should not have intercourse or douche for 48 hours before the smear. If the patient has used antibiotic vaginal creams, the exam should be delayed a month. The use of any medications, particularly birth control pills, should be noted on the request slip. For some women, a pelvic exam is an unpleasant and embarrassing procedure, and the nurse must be sensitive to the need to respect the privacy of the patient by draping procedures, etc. There are do-it-yourself-type kits for Papanicolaou tests. If the woman is to collect the sample herself, she must be taught how deep in the vagina she must go to get the specimen and how to fix it in the proper preservative. As a guide, the woman can be told that the cervical os feels like the tip of the nose. Nurses may also do Papanicolaou smears as part of a health screening program. Fisher et al. (1977) describes the role of the nurse in doing Papanicolaou smears in the general hospital setting.

Postest Nursing Implications

There are no patient restrictions after a Papanicolaou smear. If the cytology report shows atypical cells, the patient may have a colposcopy and cervical biopsy done.

COLPOSCOPY AND CERVICAL BIOPSY

Description: The colposcope or colpomicroscope is a binocular microscope with a magnifying glass and a high-intensity light source, and is used to examine the vagina and cervix. The biopsy is planned for about a week after the patient's menses because the cervix is more vascular before and after the menses. The biopsy is done after the menstrual period so there is no possibility of a pregnancy. (See the 10- to 14-day rule discussed in Chapter 1, for x-ray procedures for women of childbearing age.) The patient is prepared for a pelvic exam as described earlier. The patient is not given any local anesthetic because the cervix is sensitive to pressure but not to burning or cutting, as is the skin. The momentary pressure will be slightly uncomfortable for some patients. The biopsy site may be sealed with a silver nitrate stick or cauterized. A packing will probably be put in the vagina.
Purposes: With the colposcope, the clinician can identify areas of the cervix that appear atypical and thus, perform direct punch biopsies. It takes about 10 minutes to view the cervical epithelium and note suspicious areas. Normally, the cervix is pink. During pregnancy, the cervix becomes dusky in color. After menopause the cervix is light pink. Any secretions should be odorless and clear. The stickiness of the secretions is related to ovulation time. If abnormal areas are seen in the cervix, or if there are abnormal secretions, a cervical biopsy and/or an endocervical curettage should be done. Nurses, as primary care practitioners, may do colposcopic exams. Mulligan et al. (1975) describe the role of the nurse in a nurse-run colposcopy clinic. Endometrial biopsies may be done as part of an infertility work-up (see Chapter 9).

Posttest Nursing Implications

Often a cervical biopsy is done on an outpatient basis. If a cone biopsy is needed, the patient must be given general anesthesia. The patient should be told that she will feel some pressure and that slight bleeding is normal. The vaginal packing or tampon is left in place for several hours. Any unusual bleeding or severe abdominal pain should be reported immediately. Some spotting is expected. The patient needs to be given instructions about when intercourse can be resumed.

BREAST BIOPSY AND NEEDLE ASPIRATION

Description and Purposes: A breast biopsy or needle aspiration as diagnostic procedures for malignancies are being done more often in an outpatient setting. Many surgeons still do a breast biopsy while the patient is under a general anesthetic so that a mastectomy can be immediately done if the frozen section is positive for cancer. However, the newer trend is to wait and perform the mastectomy at a later date. Several reports have demonstrated that a short delay between biopsy and mastectomy does not adversely affect survival (Townsend, 1980). This delay gives the patient and family more time to adjust to the surgery. For a breast biopsy, the skin is prepped and the patient is draped and anesthetized in the usual manner. A small amount of tissue is incised. Either a biopsy or needle aspiration takes only a few minutes to complete and may be used to determine the need for more explorative surgery.

Pretest Nursing Implications

The set-up for the procedure is similar to that for any other local biopsy—sterile drapes and local anesthetic. The physical discomfort is minimal, but the anxiety level of the woman, or, less frequently, the man, is likely to be quite high. Although the majority of breast lumps are *not* malignant, there is always the possibility that this one may be. Roughly 80 percent of breast lumps are benign (National Cancer Institute, 1980).

Posttest Nursing Implications

The patient should be told exactly when the results will be available because the waiting time can be very difficult. If a biopsy was done, there may be a few stitches, which need to be removed. The woman should wear a supportive bra 24 hours a day until healing is completed. The nipple may have numbness for a couple of months, which can interfere with sexual arousal (Wiley, 1981).

The nurse can also make sure that the patient does know how to do self-breast exams. (See Chapter 1 for information on mammograms as screening devices for high-risk women.) Luckmann & Sorensen (1980) has excellent material on patient-teaching about breast cancer. The Department of Health and Human Services also publishes a pamphlet on breast self-examination, which can be obtained free for patient teaching.

LIVER BIOPSY

Description: A liver biopsy can be done at the patient's bedside or in a special treatment room. The skin is prepped and anesthetized. Before the biopsy needle is inserted into the liver, the patient is asked to take a deep breath and then hold the breath after an expiration. Not breathing keeps the diaphragm motionless. Also, holding the breath after an expiration leaves the diaphragm further up in the thoracic cavity than after an inspiration. (For a renal biopsy, the patient is asked to hold his breath after inspiration, which is a little easier to do.) For children or confused adults, the nose can be momentarily blocked at the end of an expiration. At the end of a cry, the child will have maximal expiration. Obviously it is much more desirable to have a quiet, cooperative patient because jerking or thrashing about can cause a tear in the liver. An uncooperative patient usually makes the procedure unsafe. The actual insertion of the needle and a collection of tissue only takes a minute or two. The entire procedure can be done in 10 or 15 minutes. When the needle is withdrawn, a pressure dressing is applied to the area.

Purposes: A liver biopsy may be useful in determining the exact nature of liver pathology, such as tumors, cysts, or cirrhosis. A sonogram (Chapter 4) or a liver scan (Chapter 3) gives the physician valuable information about the exact area to biopsy.

Pretest Nursing Implications

The patient must have coagulation tests (PT, PTT, and platelet counts) done before the liver biopsy. A hematocrit (Hct) will also be done as a baseline assessment. For a liver biopsy, the general rule is that the prothrombin time (PT) activity should be over 50 percent and not more than three seconds over the control in time. The platelets should be above 100,000 cu/mm (Boyer & Oehlberg, 1977). Because a diseased liver may be unable to manufacture prothrombin in normal amounts, vitamin K may be ordered in an attempt to raise the PT percentage and decrease the time in seconds. See Corbett (1982) for a discussion on laboratory tests for prothrombin and the relationship to liver disease and vitamin K.

The patient is usually kept on n.p.o. status for about six hours before the test. Fasting makes the liver less congested and the biliary ducts less turgid. Fasting also prevents any vomiting if complications occur. The patient is usually not given any sedation, but some sedation may be needed in selected cases. Baseline vital signs are taken, and the patient is given a chance to practice holding the breath after an expiration.

Posttest Nursing Implications

Preventing and Detecting Bleeding. The patient is turned on his or her right side for one to four hours. Bed rest may continue for 8 to 12 hours or longer. A sandbag may be used to apply pressure to the area. It is important to check the dressing for any bleeding, but a pressure dressing should *not* be removed to look for bleeding. Usually serious bleeding will be internal, and thus, it is not detected by visual inspection. Patients can bleed to death from a liver biopsy, therefore, vital signs are checked frequently, as with any invasive procedure. Food may be withheld until it is certain that the patient is not having any immediate complications. An eight-hour posttest hematocrit (Hct) may be done to assess for any blood loss. Even a slight drop in the Hct should be called to the physician's attention.

Assessing and Preventing Other Complications. In addition to hemorrhage and shock, other complications that can occur from a liver biopsy include bile peritonitis, pneumothorax, or perforation of an abdominal organ (e.g., the colon). Any pain in the abdomen or any dyspnea calls for a thorough physical assessment of the thorax and abdomen. Slight pain at the biopsy site can be expected as the local anesthetic wears off. The patient may be kept on bedrest for an entire 24 hours or longer if there are any complications. The patient should be cautioned not to cough or strain because this can increase intraabdominal pressure. The day after the biopsy, the patient can resume most activities, but should not do strenuous activities or heavy lifting for a week or two.

RENAL BIOPSIES

Description: The renal biopsy is usually done in a treatment room close to the ultrasound or x-ray department because the insertion of the needle is monitored by fluoroscopy or scanning. Renal biopsies can also be done with a cystoscope, using a brush inserted up into the ureter to get a fragment of renal tissue (Gittes, 1978). The brush technique with a cystoscope requires general anesthesia so is done in the operating room. A renal biopsy, done under a local, may be done through a skin puncture (closed biopsy) or through a small skin incision (open biopsy). The skin is prepped and anesthesized as usual. The patient is usually not given any sedation, but the use of drugs will not interfere with the procedure. The patient is asked to take a breath and hold it while the needle is being inserted to obtain the biopsy. Only a very small piece of tissue is obtained. When the needle is withdrawn a pressure dressing is applied to the area, and the patient is transported back to the nursing unit.

Purposes: Renal biopsies are most helpful in diagnosing diseases that alter the structure of the glomeruli (Fennel, 1975). Only the cortex is biopsied, not the medulla. Renal biopsies may also determine the exact nature of a mass, which could be a tumor, clot, or stone. Renal biopsies may be done periodically to evaluate and monitor the course of chronic renal disease, such as the nephrotic syndrome.

Pretest Nursing Implications

Preparation is similar to that for a liver biopsy in that coagulation studies (PT, PTT, and platelet count) must be done, vital signs taken for a baseline, and hematocrit (Hct) done. In addition, the patient should have an urinalysis and an intravenous pyelogram done (Chapter 1) to determine that there are two functioning kidneys. The patient is usually allowed food and fluids before the procedure, but this should be checked. As mentioned before, sedation does not affect the test and might be needed if the patient is very anxious even after optimal preparation. The patient should be told approximately how long he or she will be in the radiology or ultrasound department and what the aftercare will be.

Posttest Nursing Implications

The patient is usually instructed to remain relatively motionless for four hours. A sandbag may be placed on the biopsy site. Bedrest may be continued for 24 hours. If a piece of artery is discovered in the biopsy tissue, the bedrest may be prolonged. Vital signs and dressing check routines are done. A hematocrit is usually ordered eight hours after the procedure.

Observing Fluid Intake and Output. During the first 24 hours, urine is collected in separate cups and left in the bathroom so any hematuria can be monitored. The timing of each specimen should be marked on the cup. Some urine may also be sent to the laboratory for microscopic examination. Microscopic hematuria occurs in about half of the cases, and a few cases will show some gross hematuria (Fennell, 1975). There are dipsticks for detecting occult hematuria, but these are not as sensitive as a microscopic examination. (See Corbett (1982) Chapter 13 on guaiac tests and Chapter 2 on urinalysis.) The patient should have a large intake of fluids, up to 2000 ml for an adult, to promote urinary function.

Patient Teaching to Avoid Other Complications. The major complication from a renal biopsy is hemorrhage. Any severe jolt to the retro-peritoneal area can cause bleeding, even several days after the biopsy. The patient should be instructed to avoid strenuous activities or heavy lifting for several days. The patient should also be told to report any flank pain, gross hematuria, or signs of dizziness or weakness. Infection can occur after a biopsy so the patient's temperature should be routinely checked for a day after the biopsy. The patient should report any burning on urination.

Questions

1. Which of the following invasive procedures is not done on an outpatient basis?

a. Thoracentesis or pleural tap
b. Lumbar puncture
c. Bone marrow aspiration and biopsy
d. Liver biopsy

2. Which of the following nursing actions is *not routine* in preparing a patient for any invasive diagnostic procedure to be done at the bedside?

a. Withholding all medications, food, and liquids
b. Helping prepare the patient on ways to cope with pain or discomfort
c. Checking to make sure the specific tray needed for the procedure is available
d. Taking a baseline blood pressure and leaving the blood pressure cuff on the arm

3. Epinephrine may be added to a local anesthetic, such as lidocaine (Xylocaine), to

a. Increase the duration of the local anesthetic
b. Decrease the allergic effects of the anesthetic
c. Decrease local bleeding
d. Both a and c

4. Timmy, age 4, must have a bone marrow aspiration done. Which of the following actions by the nurse would be the *least* helpful in preparing Timmy for this invasive procedure?

a. Letting Timmy play with replicas of some of the equipment
b. Telling Timmy how he can help during the procedure
c. Explaining the reason for the procedure
d. Telling Timmy briefly about how the procedure will feel (i.e., some pain)

5. Mr. Fox has just had a lumbar puncture done. Which of these factors seems to be the most significant in preventing Mr. Fox from developing a "spinal headache"?

a. Keeping Mr. Fox flat in bed for 6 to 12 hours after the procedure
b. Keeping Mr. Fox on n.p.o. status for two to three hours after the procedure

c. The use of a small-sized needle for the lumbar puncture
d. The use of prophylactic analgesics after the procedure

6. The physician thinks Mr. Fox may have bacterial meningitis. Which of the following decreases in the CSF when there is a bacterial infection and is *routinely* done as part of the CSF analysis?

a. Glucose
b. Lymphocytes
c. Protein
d. Chlorides

7. Which of the following nursing actions is not appropriate for Mrs. Sangria who just had a thoracentesis done? Four hundred ml of clear fluid was obtained from the right pleural space.

a. Encouraging extra fluids orally to rehydrate Mrs. Sangria
b. Assessing the thorax for diminished breath sounds
c. Positioning Mrs. Sangria on her left side for one hour after the thoracentesis
d. Reporting any symptoms of blood in the sputum (hemoptysis) or shortness of breath (dyspnea)

8. Mr. Heppy is to have an abdominal paracentesis done this morning. Which of the following nursing actions is *not* routine for this diagnostic procedure?

a. Making sure that the patient's bladder is empty
b. Using sterile equipment for the procedure
c. Helping the patient assume a comfortable side lying position for the procedure
d. Letting the patient eat as tolerated

9. Procedures done for a gastric analysis may include all the following *except*

a. Administration of atropine to dry up secretions before the test
b. Insertion of a nasogastric tube that stays in the stomach for the duration of the test
c. Administration of betazole hydrochloride (Histalog) to stimulate gastric secretions
d. Collection of samples for detecting Papanicolaou cells and the presence of acid-fast bacillus

10. The latest American Cancer Society recommendation (1980) on the frequency of Papanicolaou smears for women age 20 to 40 is that after two yearly Papanicolaou smears are negative, the Papanicolaou smear should be done

a. Annually
b. Every two years
c. Every three years
d. Only for high-risk individuals

11. Mr. Cronkite is to have a liver biopsy done today. Which of the following nursing actions is *not* appropriate in preparing Mr. Cronkite for the liver biopsy?

a. Have him practice holding his breath after an expiration

b. Keep him on n.p.o. status before the test

c. Explain that a local anesthetic will be used to eliminate the pain

d. Explain that he can resume normal activities as soon as the biopsy is finished and his vital signs are stable

12. Mr. Ralph has just returned from the radiology department where he had a closed-renal biopsy done with a local anesthetic. Which of the nursing actions is *not* appropriate?

a. Keep Mr. Ralph as motionless as possible on bedrest for four hours

b. Save all urine in one container for a 24-hour urine sample

c. Administer the ordered analgesic for pain at the biopsy site

d. Encourage fluid intake to 2000 ml if possible

REFERENCES

American Cancer Society. ''Report on the Cancer-Related Health Checkup.'' New York: American Cancer Society, Inc. (February 8 1980).

American College of Obstetricians and Gynecologists. ''Cancer Test Controversy'' reported in *Maternal Child Nursing* 5: 430 (November/December 1980).

Barber, J. et al. *Adult and Child Care: A Client Approach to Nursing*. St. Louis: C. V. Mosby, 1977.

Beck, M. ''Preparing Your Patient Physically For an Esophagogastroduodenoscopy.'' *Nursing 81* 11: 88–96 (February 1981).

Beckemeyer, P. & Bahr, J. ''Helping Toddlers and Pre-Schoolers Cope While Suturing Their Minor Lacerations.'' *Maternal Child Nursing* 5: 326–330 (September/October 1980).

Boyer, C. & Oehlberg, S. ''Interpretation and Clinical Relevance of Liver Function Tests.'' *Nursing Clinics of North America* 12: 275–285 (June 1977).

Cohen, S. et al. ''Radioimmunoassay of Myelin Basic Protein in Spinal Fluid.'' *New England Journal of Medicine* 295: 1455–1457 (December 23, 1976).

Corbett, J. V. *Laboratory Tests in Nursing Practice*. Norwalk, CT: Appleton-Century-Crofts, 1982.

Cosgriff, J. *An Atlas of Diagnostic and Therapeutic Procedures for Emergency Personnel*. Philadelphia: J. B. Lippincott, 1978.

Fennell, S. ''Percutaneous Renal Biopsy.'' *American Journal of Nursing* 75: 1292–1294 (August 1975).

Fisher, D. et al. ''Nurse-Run Pap Smear as Hospital Screening.'' *Connecticut Medicine* 41: 143–145 (March 1977).

Fisher, D. ''Abdominal Paracentesis for Malignant Ascites.'' *Archives Internal Medicine* 139: 235 (February 1979).

Gittes, R. ''Retrograde Renal and Ureteral Brush Biopsy.'' *American Journal of Nursing* 78: 410–412 (March 1978).

Johnson, J. et al. "Altering Children's Distress Behavior During Cast Removal." *Nursing Research* 24: 404–410 (November/December 1975).

Johnson, J. "Sensory Information, Instruction in a Coping Strategy and Recovery from Surgery." *Research in Nursing and Health* 1: 4–17 (April 1978).

Johnson, J. E. & Rice, V. H. "Sensory and Distress Components of Pain: Implications for Study of Clinical Pain." *Nursing Research* 23: 203–209 (May/June 1974).

Koepke, J. *Guide to Clinical Laboratory Diagnosis,* 2nd ed. Norwalk, CT: Appleton-Century-Crofts, 1980.

Luckmann, J. & Sorenson, K. *Medical-Surgical Nursing: A Psychophysiologic Approach,* 2nd ed. Philadelphia: W. B. Saunders, 1980.

Miller, B. & Keane, C. *Encyclopedia and Dictionary of Medicine, Nursing and Allied Health,* 2 ed. Philadelphia: W. B. Saunders, 1978.

Markus, S. "Taking the Fear out of Bone Marrow Examinations." *Nursing 81:* 64–67 (April 1981).

Mulligan, C. et al. "Screening for Cervical Cancer." *American Journal of Nursing* 75: 1343–1344 (August 1975).

National Cancer Institute. *Breast Self-Examination.* U.S. Department of Health and Human Services, NIH Publication #80-649 (August 1980).

Petito, F. & Plum, F. "The Lumbar Puncture." *New England Journal of Medicine* 290: 225–226 (January 24, 1974).

Phipps, W. et al. *Medical-Surgical Nursing: Concepts and Clinical Practice.* St. Louis: C. V. Mosby Co., 1979.

Pidgeon, V. "Characteristics of Children's Thinking and Implications for Health Teaching." *Maternal-Child Nursing Journal* 6: 1–7 (Spring 1977).

Rank, D. et al. "Evaluation of Abnormal Cervical Cytology." *Obstetrics and Gynecology* 49: 581–586 (May 1977).

Sculley, R. E. "Normal Reference Values." *New England Journal of Medicine* 302: 48 (January 3, 1980).

Shetler, M. & Bartos, H. "Spinal and Peritoneal Taps." *RN* 44: 50–53 (January 1981).

Taylor, J. & Ballenger, S. *Neurological Dysfunctions and Nursing Intervention.* New York: McGraw-Hill, 1980.

Townsend, C. "Breast Lumps: Diagnostic Techniques." *Ciba Clinical Symposia* 32: 22–24 (February 1980).

Tucker, S. et al. *Patient Care Standards.* St. Louis: C. V. Mosby, 1980.

Wiley, K. "Post-Biopsy Care." *American Journal of Nursing* 81: 1553–1662 (September 1981).

CHAPTER SEVEN

Stress Tests and Cardiac Catheterizations

Objectives

1. Describe the general purposes of stress testing (exercise treadmill electrocardiographs) for healthy individuals and for those with some degree of heart disease.
2. Explain what nurses should teach patients about stress testing.
3. Describe appropriate nursing interventions before and after stress tests.
4. Explain how stress test results are used to plan activity levels.
5. Compare the purposes and procedures of right-sided and left-sided cardiac catheterizations.
6. Describe appropriate nursing interventions before and after cardiac catheterization.
7. Identify expected effects of medications used before and during cardiac catheterizations.

Chapters 5 and 6 have given basic information about noninvasive and invasive testing, respectively. This chapter discusses stress testing, a noninvasive test, which, unlike other noninvasive tests, is not risk free. Although stress testing is fairly common, it is not always well understood by nurses or the general community. Even if nurses are not involved in stress testing procedures, they should be able to explain the test and the needed precautions to patients and their families. Stress tests can be very dangerous if not conducted properly. Nurses help prepare patients for the tests, sometimes help administer the test, and more often are involved in follow-up programs for cardiac rehabilitation (see Janz & Lampman, 1981 and Sivarajan & Halpenny, 1979).

The second test covered in this chapter, cardiac catheterization, is a sophisticated invasive cardiac procedure. In the past few years, as cardiac catheterization has become a common practice in most medical centers, many nurses have become involved in preparing patients for cardiac catheterizations and caring for patients during the recovery phase.

The cardiac catheterization laboratory not only requires elaborate equipment, it also requires a team of highly skilled clinicians. A cardiologist, trained to do cardiac catheterizations, heads a team comprised of various technicians, who are highly skilled in using the laboratory's monitoring equipment. Registered nurses are sometimes part of a cardiac catheterization team. In addition to being an assistant during the procedure, the nurse may also help prepare the patient for the procedure and do a follow-up assessment. (Several of the references used in this chapter were written by nurses who function as part of a cardiac catheterization team.)

STRESS TESTING

Description: The forerunner of the modern heart stress test was the Master's two-step test, which involved stepping up and down on a 20-cm platform 30 times a minute while an ECG recorded the effect of the stress on the heart (Miller, 1978). The more modern stress test is done in a cardiology laboratory, which is set up to monitor blood pressure, ECG, and sometimes oxygen consumption while the patient exercises by walking on a treadmill. The treadmill is speeded up at intervals and the pitch is changed to determine the exercise tolerance of the individual. The test is continued until a predetermined end-point has been obtained or the patient shows signs of undue fatigue. A stationary exercise bicycle called a bicycle ergometer, which is portable and cheaper than a treadmill can be used. However, it is not as easy to standardize the results because many people develop thigh muscle fatigue before they reach their maximum heart rate.

When assessing exercise tolerance in cardiac patients, a physician must be present so the test can be stopped if certain clinical symptoms or dangerous arrhythmias develop. For a healthy person undergoing exercise tolerance testing, a physician or qualified delegate can observe the patient's response while on the treadmill. A certification examination for stress exercise testing is given by the American College of Sports Medicine (Sivarajan & Halpenny, 1979). Nurses must realize that stress testing can be a dangerous procedure if not handled properly. Only qualified people should conduct the tests. The American Heart Association (1979) has excellent information on quality control for operation of an exercise tolerance laboratory.

Before beginning the test, the patient must be told exactly what to expect and that he or she can stop the test at any time, but the test is of greater value if the exercise is continued until a certain predetermined level is obtained. The predetermined levels are arbitrarily set, based on the patient's age and expected response to a certain level of exercise. Tables show the usual maximal heart rate for different ages. The target heart rate to be achieved may be up to 85 percent of the estimate for the maximal heart rate for a certain age. For example, an untrained person age 40 may have a maximal heart rate of 189; thus, the recommended target heart rate would be 161 (American Heart Association, 1979).

The patient is connected to the apparatus necessary to monitor ECG, blood pressure readings, and if oxygen consumption is done, a mouthpiece is used. Baseline measurements are taken in advance, and the physician does a brief physical assessment to clear the patient for the test.

After the patient has a chance to practice walking on the treadmill, the test is begun. The ECG is constantly monitored and oxygen consumption, blood pressure, and heart rate are recorded every three minutes.

During the test, clinicians assess for symptoms, such as vertigo, extreme dyspnea, pallor, or signs of exhaustion. Depending on the ECG reading and other circumstances, the patient may be allowed to continue with mild or moderate angina, but severe angina necessitates an abrupt end of the test. Leg fatigue or severe pain in the calves of the leg (claudication) may also necessitate a halt of the test.

Other reasons to stop the test would be (Janz & Lampman, 1981):

1. Fall of systolic blood pressure of 22 mmHg
2. Marked S–T segment depression
3. Ventricular tachycardia
4. Heart block, second or third degree
5. Atrial fibrillation
6. Paroxysmal atrial tachycardia.

Some people do have occasional ectopic beats with exercise so a few premature atrial contractions (PACs) or even premature ventricular contractions (PVCs) are not indications to stop the test if there is no clinical evidence of a change in cardiac output. (See Chapter 5 for a detailed discussion on common types of arrhythmias and clinical assessment for changes in cardiac output.)

Note that a thallium scan may be done in conjunction with a stress test. Thallium scans may be particularly useful for a patient with multivessel coronary disease (Smeets, 1981). (See Chapter 3 for a discussion on cardiac imaging with thallium. The patient receives thallium intravenously.)

Purposes:

Assessing Exercise Tolerance

When planning exercise programs, stress tests are done to evaluate the exercise tolerance of an individual. The information from a stress test is useful in planning a graduated exercise program for an individual. Even for people without cardiac disease, a stress test may be used to evaluate cardiovascular function to help a person train effectively.

Stress tests are even more necessary in presumably healthy individuals with risk factors for coronary disease, such as hypertension, hyperlipidemia, or cigarette smoking (American Heart Association, 1975). Individuals with known heart disease are also evaluated for exercise tolerance. For example, a patient with an uncomplicated myocardial infarction may have a stress test ten days to two weeks after the infarction (Janz & Lampman, 1981). Stress testing may also be used to assess the exercise capacity of a patient with pulmonary disease.

Computation of Energy Units: Metabolic Equivalent Levels. Metabolic equivalent level (MET) is the energy expenditure at rest, equivalent to approximately 3.5 ml O_2 per kg/body weight per minute. The metabolic equivalent level is determined by dividing the patient's exercise oxygen consumption by the resting oxygen consumption. Tables can be used to determine an individual's total capability in terms of METs. The American Heart Association (1975) has published charts that show the metabolic equivalent of various activities. For example, level walking at two miles an hour, takes about 2 to 3 METs, walking four miles an hour takes 5 to 6 METs, and running six miles per hour takes 10 METs. The charts also show the approximate metabolic cost of many occupational and recreational activities in terms of METs.

Assessing Coronary Ischemia and Arrhythmias

Stress testing is also used to help diagnose chest pain or arrhythmias triggered by physical stress. The stress test may allow diagnosis of early ischemia heart disease, undetected by a resting ECG. (The test can also demonstrate if there is a correlation between clinical symptoms and certain arrhythmias.)

The characteristic sign of myocardial ischemia is a depressed S-T segment. The changes in the S-T segment must be carefully analyzed by a cardiologist. Some patients have a drop in the S-T segment when standing or hyperventilating; thus, these factors and others must be considered so as not to make a false diagnosis of coronary artery insufficiency (Wenger et al., 1980). A cardiac catheterization, discussed later in this chapter, may be needed to determine the extent and exact location of atherosclerotic plaques in the coronary arteries.

Drugs, such as nitroglycerin, may be given during the test to evaluate their effectiveness for angina. Nitroglycerine can cause considerable improvement in exercise tolerance. Nitroglycerin causes some venous pooling and thus a reduction of left ventricular volume and some reduction of arterial pressure (Simoons, 1981).

Pretest Nursing Implications

Obtaining Informed Consent. Although a stress test can yield valuable information, it is not risk free, even when patients have been carefully screened. The exercise, which is equal in stress to walking briskly or running up a steep hill, can cause severe arrhythmias, a myocardial infarction, or a stroke in susceptible individuals. Most authorities quote a mortality rate of about 0.01 percent or one death in every 10,000 patients tested. Because of the risk of morbidity and even mortality, the patient must sign an informed consent after the physician explains the benefits versus the risks. The nurse can reassure the patient that trained personnel and emergency equipment will be available in the laboratory to deal with any complications that may occur.

Many institutions have written information about stress tests, including the risks and benefits of the test. One such patient information sheet stresses, ''You should not feel that you are being pressured or persuaded to have the test if you feel at all uncomfortable about it'' (Kaiser Permanente Medical Center, 1981). People should be given *time* to digest verbal and written information and then make an informed decision. (See Chapter 6 for more about the role of the nurse as the advocate for the patient who is having invasive tests or tests which can cause complications.)

Limiting Food and Fluid Intake. The patient should eat a light meal a couple of hours before the test. Some clinicians prefer that the person have no beverages containing caffeine while others allow one cup of coffee or tea before the test. Milk or other foods, which may cause nausea during exercise, should be avoided. The person should be adequately hydrated before the test.

Administering Medications. If the patient is on diuretics, assessment of the serum potassium level is done before the exercise test. Hypokalemia, often a side effect of diuretics, predisposes the person to arrhythmias. If patients are taking digitalis, they are usually not considered candidates for stress testing, but this is an individual medical decision. Nitroglycerin or other vasodilators are not given before the test, unless the test is being done to evaluate the efficiency of the medications. Pain medications, even aspirin, may invalidate the test. The nurse must confer with the doctor to see what medications are permissible before the test. Patients need clear instructions on which routine medications are to be continued and which are to be withheld.

Clothing Needs. Comfortable *walking* shoes are a must for the test. Bedroom slippers, sandals, or high-heeled shoes are unsatisfactory. Rubber-soled shoes provide the best grip on the treadmill.

Men strip to the waist so electrodes can be applied to the chest area. Women can wear a bra and a hospital gown or blouse, which opens in the front. Pants, skirts, or trousers should be loose and comfortable. Constricting clothing and nylon fabrics are to be avoided. Hair should be arranged off the face, and any bothersome jewelry should be removed.

Resting before the Test. A good night's sleep before the test is essential so undue fatigue is not a factor in the results. Relaxation exercises before the test may be beneficial. The patient goes through some warming up exercises and cooling down exercises in the laboratory. No other diagnostic procedures or tests should be scheduled on the same day.

Posttest Nursing Implications

Assessing Vital Signs. The patient remains in the cardiology laboratory until vital signs are normal. To ensure that baseline levels have returned, ECG tracings are taken at various intervals. Very rarely, the patient may need to be monitored for several hours because of an arrhythmia or other complication. If the patient returns to a nursing unit, vital signs are checked at certain intervals to assess the patient's stability.

Promoting Rest and Relaxation. An outpatient may be allowed to drive home, depending on the circumstances. After the test, the patient should rest for the remainder of the day. A shower should not be taken for a few hours because the warm water and standing may cause vasodilation. If the patient's performance level was low, the nurse can help the person ventilate his or her feelings of dejection.

Resuming Food and Fluids. Depending on the level of exertion, the person may be thirsty, and fluids should be provided. As with other exercise, hunger may be abated for a while, but diet can be normally resumed.

Planning Follow-Ups. The MET levels, discussed earlier, can be helpful in gauging the expected exercise capability of the person. An individualized exercise program is planned on the basis of the various results of the stress testing. An ideal exercise plan is one which helps the person achieve the target heart rate for 30 minutes three times a week. Target heart rates may be up to 85 percent of the person's maximum heart rate. The American Heart Association (1975) has detailed guidelines for exercise prescriptions. Whatever the length and type of exercise prescribed by the physician, it is important that the patient also understand the importance of warm-up and cooling-down exercises. Janz & Lampman (1981) and Sivarjan & Halpenny (1981) both discuss the role of the nurse in conducting exercise programs.

If the stress test was done to evaluate angina and possible coronary ischemia, more diagnostic tests may be ordered by the physician. For example, the patient may need instructions about cardiac catheterizations, discussed next.

CARDIAC CATHETERIZATION

Description: A cardiac catheterization is done under local anesthetic because the patient needs to cooperate by doing some deep breathing and coughing maneuvers. The patient may also be asked to do bicycle-type leg exercises to see the effect of stress on cardiac function and coronary blood flow. (Small children are catheterized under general anesthesia.) Depending on the information needed, a catheter may be inserted into a vein for a study of the right side of the heart or into an artery (usually the femoral artery) for a study of the left side of the heart. The catheter for cardiac catheterization is a flexible hollow tube about 2 mm wide—the thickness of a ballpoint pen refill. The tube is 100 cm, or 40 inches, long. For a left-sided catheterization, an artery is punctured by a short stubby needle and a guide wire is inserted. The catheter slides over the guide wire into the artery. The guide wire makes it possible to guide the catheter through the left atrium into the left ventricle. Fluoroscopy is used to view the catheter—the room must be darkened. (See Chapter 1 for a discussion on fluoroscopy.) For a right-sided catheterization, a vein is used, and the catheter is threaded via the vena cava into the right atrium and right ventricle.

A transseptal technique uses a small needle inserted in the right side of the heart, which is gently maneuvered through the septum to get pressure readings and blood samples from the left side of the heart. In some cases of aortic stenosis, the heart's valve cannot be crossed in the usual manner, and a transseptal technique is needed.

After the pressures and readings and blood samples are obtained, a catheter is threaded into the coronary artery and a radiopaque dye is inserted to outline the coronary arteries. This dye, diatrizoale (Hyopaque) contains iodine (see Chapter 1 for the precautions when dye with iodine is used for a diagnostic procedure). During the passage of the dye, the room is darkened so that the motion can be observed on the fluoroscope screen. Movies (cineography) may also be taken of the flow of the dye.

The entire procedure of a left-sided and right-sided cardiac catheterization takes about one to two hours, depending on the findings. However, patients may not need all the different aspects done. For example, an adolescent with a valve defect may not have studies done of the coronary arteries.

Because cardiac catheterization is an elaborate procedure requiring a specialized laboratory set-up, it is not done in small hospitals or clinics.

Purposes: As mentioned earlier in this chapter, the stress test may be a preliminary test before cardiac catheterization. Cardiac catheterization is used when noninvasive forms of cardiac diagnostic tests—such as echocardiograms (Chapter 4), ECG, phonocardiograms (Chapter 5), and radionuclide scans (Chapter 3)—have not provided enough diagnostic information. As with any invasive procedure, there is a certain amount of risk for the patient, and if less complicated, less risky, and less costly procedures will suffice, they are preferred.

Cardiac catheterization is often needed to confirm the need for heart surgery. For example, the need for a coronary bypass procedure is assessed by cardiac catheterization, which demonstrates the lack of coronary perfusion. Cardiac catheterization also defines the exact type of other cardiac problems, especially congenital heart defects. Cardiac catheterization can also determine the severity of the heart disease and evaluate the progress of the patient after medical or surgical interventions.

Conventional cardiac catheterization measures the pressures and calculates the flows in the various chambers of the heart and "great" vessels. Blood samples are obtained to measure dilutions of dye and oxygen and carbon dioxide values. Radiopaque dye is used to take x-rays and fluoroscopy of the heart and vessels. More advanced procedures such as the His-bundle ECG or coronary sinus lactate determination are discussed in specialty texts, such as Wenger et al. (1980).

Pretest Nursing Implications

Checking the Chart. The patient's chart will contain the results of other diagnostic tests, such as coagulation studies, hematocrit, etc. In addition, vital signs and other baseline data are charted as for other invasive procedures (see Chapter 6). The precatheterization physical stability of the patient must be assessed and documented.

Although the risks of major complications, such as a myocardial infarction or cerebral vascular accident, are slight, they sometimes occur with a catheterization. Thus, the patient must sign a consent form that lists the possible complications, including such things as the possibility of a loss of a limb or cardiac arrest (Cogen, 1976). Obviously, the individual's physician must explain the possibility of such risks in relationship to the potential greater benefits of the procedure.

Patient-Teaching. A nurse from the cardiac catheterization lab or from the general unit should reinforce the explanation of the cardiac catherization procedure. Most cardiac catheterization laboratories have patient information booklets, which describe the procedure and answer common questions that patients may have about the preparation for the test. For example, Kaiser Permanente Medical Centers in Northern California have a booklet that explains not only the catheterization procedure, but also why the patient must come to the San Francisco facility and be admitted to the hospital for the procedure. The booklet even contains a map of the medical center to help the referred patient find the hospital and parking lot. The patient checks in the night before or arrives the day of the procedure. Some institutions use audio–visual material to explain the cardiac catheterization procedure. This can be done the morning of the exam. Studies have not shown whether it is more or less effective to have patients actually visit the cardiac lab before the procedure (Edwards & Payton, 1976). Without adequate preparation, viewing the "cath lab'' may be anxiety-producing. Teasley (1982) has suggested a check list for teaching the patient about the procedure, followed by viewing the laboratory—if feasible.

Explaining the Pain and Discomfort from Cardiac Catheterization. Disch (1979) has found some patients experience much discomfort during a cardiac catheterization, while others do not. The anxiety level of the patient seems to be an important factor. Certainly, the idea of a catheter entering one's heart is a frightening idea. The nurse should explain to the patient that he or she may experience a little discomfort so that he or she does not imagine the worse. Because the positioning of the catheter may cause a rapid or irregular pulse, the patient may feel his or her heart ''flip-flop'' or race. Therefore, it may be comforting for the patient to know that arrhythmias are rather common during the threading of the catheter and usually disappear without treatment. The patient should be told that there will be constant monitoring for serious arrhythmias and that emergency equipment and drugs will be present for immediate use.

Another discomfort is a venous or, even more so, an arterial puncture. A local anesthetic is used before the arterial puncture, but there is usually some pain associated with the procedure. Needles in general are very unpleasant for some people. (See Chapter 6 on ways nurses can help prepare patients for momentary pain.) The injection of the dye may be a source of pain or discomfort for some patients, because of a metallic taste, a warm feeling, or a more intense ''rush'' from the dye. (The symptoms of an allergic reaction can occur, but this is not common, see Chapter 1.) Another discomfort may be the length of time the patient must lie relatively still on the table—this may be very taxing for some patients. Nevertheless, the discomforts should be explained to the patient.

Physical Preparation of Patient. The patient's groin, used for the femoral puncture, should be shaved. This may be done on the unit or in the laboratory. Depending on the policy of the institution, the patient may be allowed clear liquids or kept on n.p.o. status. Fluids may be withheld because of the danger of aspiration if an emergency occurs (Finesilver, 1980). The patient should void and empty his or her bowels, if possible, because the procedure is a long one. The patient is transported to the laboratory by stretcher. A hospital gown is worn. Glasses can be worn, as well as a watch because the patient will be awake. Dentures are left in place because they may be needed if the patient is to do any breathing exercises with a mouthpiece. Hearing aides should be worn if needed. The patient's chart should note the presence of a hearing difficulty or any communication problems.

Use of Medications before the Procedure. Routine medications are usually not withheld, but this should be checked with the cardiologist. Certain drugs, such as long-term anticoagulants, are usually contraindicated before the procedure because of the risk of bleeding. Thus, if a patient has been on coumarin (Coumadin), this must be evaluated by the physician. The premedications differ from institution to institution. Atropine may be given to prevent bradycardia. Atropine is an anticholinergic drug so it decreases the vagal effect from the manipulation of the catheter. Some cardiologists prefer no sedation for patients. Others routinely order a sedative, such as hydroxine (Vistaril). Antihistamines or a cortisone preparation may be ordered for patients, who are allergy-prone. Test doses of the contrast medium or dye may be done, too. During the procedure the patient may be given vasodilators, such as nitroglycerin, to promote arterial dilation. Pain medications, other than a local anesthetic, are not routine before or during the procedure. An intravenous is usually started in the laboratory, not before.

Posttest Nursing Implications

Routine Assessments. Vital signs are checked the same as for other invasive procedures. Arrhythmias usually occur during the procedure, not afterward, but an *apical* pulse should be part of the assessment each time the patient's vital signs are taken. If there is any arrhythmia, the patient may need to be monitored for a time (see Chapter 5 on monitoring). An intravenous line will be kept open (k/o rate) if arrhythmias have persisted.

Limiting Activity. The length of bedrest will depend on whether the procedure was left-sided, right-sided, or both. Bedrest for an arterial entry may be six to eight hours or longer. Some institutions routinely require strict bedrest until the next day (Teasley, 1982). With a venous entry bedrest may be only a few hours. The patient can turn from side to side while on bedrest, but the extremity used for the arterial puncture should not be moved for several hours.

Noting Differences in Arterial and Venous Puncture Sites. Because more than one entry site may be used, the nurse needs to check for more than one bandaged area, postcatheterization. Occasionally, a cutdown may be done to find the vessel for the catheter. If so, the patient will have skin sutures at the cutdown site.

A sandbag may be kept on the arterial puncture site. The outside of the pressure dressing should be checked for any bleeding or hematoma formation. The pulses distal to the arterial puncture site should be checked and compared with the uninvolved site for a thrombus in the artery. Spasms of the artery can also cause diminished arterial flow. The venous site is less likely to have any serious complications. Phlebitis (inflammation of the vein) can develop later and may be relieved by warm compresses (Luckmann & Sorensen, 1980).

Resuming Fluids and Food. The patient can eat and drink as soon as he or she desires. An adequate intake of fluids is needed to help with the excretion of the dye. Patients can have delayed allergic reactions to the iodine dye so the nurse must keep this in mind when assessing any pain or discomfort (see Chapter 1 on radiopaque dyes).

Relieving Discomfort. Back pain from the positioning is common, and a backrub may be very helpful. Mild analgesics may be needed for pain at the puncture site. Pain distal to the puncture site is not expected and could mean an embolus to the extremity.

Patients undergoing catheterization usually exhibit some of the following symptoms: fatigue, dyspnea on exertion, edema, paroxysmal nocturnal dyspnea (PND), or angina (Strong, 1977). Nurses need to know what symptoms were present before catheterization so new symptoms can be noted and called to the physician's attention. New symptoms should not be masked by pain medication.

Assessing for Cardiac Tamponade and Other Complications. In addition to arrhythmias, embolisms, and infarctions, cardiac tamponade can occur after a cardiac catheterization (Tucker, 1980). Bleeding into the pericardial sac causes reduced cardiac output, as the heart is compressed in the pericardial sac. Symptoms of cardiac tamponade include anxiety, tachypnea, distended neck veins (when the patient sits forward), muffled heart sounds, narrowing pulse pressure, and a paradoxic pulse. In order to detect a paradoxic pulse, the nurse must take the systolic blood pressure during inspiration and expiration, noting if the systolic is less during inspiration. A difference of more than 10 mm Hg in the two is evidence of a paradoxic pulse. One easy way to detect a paradoxic pulse is to ask the patient to hold his or her breath after you take the first systolic reading (Kinnebrew, 1981). Any questionable symptoms or significant change in vital signs should be immediately called to the attention of the physician. Although cardiac tamponade and other complications are unlikely after a cardiac catheterization, they can occur, and the prudent nurse is always alert for adverse reactions after all invasive tests.

Questions

1. Stress tests are done for all the following *except*

   a. Assessing the location of any myocardial ischemia
   b. Evaluating post myocardial infarction exercise tolerance
   c. Evaluating effectiveness of vasodilators for myocardial ischemia
   d. Assessing the relationship of arrhythmias to stress level

2. Mrs. Dunbar, age 48, is scheduled for a stress test tomorrow because she has had some heart palpitations while exercising. She asks the clinic nurse about the procedure. The nurse would be correct in informing Mrs. Dunbar that

   a. Blood pressures, oxygen consumption, and heart rate will be monitored during the test
   b. A treadmill will be adjusted to decreasing and increasing speeds during the test
   c. If Mrs. Dunbar has any angina, the test will stop
   d. Patients must be admitted to the hospital in preparation for the test

3. Mr. Faber has been scheduled for a stress test in the cardiology laboratory for tomorrow morning. He had an uncomplicated myocardial infarction two weeks ago. Which of the following nursing interventions is most appropriate in preparing Mr. Faber for the test?

   a. Reassuring him that there are no risks from the test
   b. Keeping him on n.p.o. status before the test
   c. Giving him nitroglycerin tablets, if needed before the test
   d. Asking his family to bring him walking shoes for the test

4. Mr. Faber's stress test demonstrated that his metabolic equivalent level (MET) was 7–8. The MET is useful in determining

a. Surgical procedures needed
b. Activity programs
c. Type of medications needed
d. Dietary needs

5. Procedures done as part of a cardiac catheterization may include all *except*

a. Fluoroscopy to guide the placement of the catheter
b. Arterial puncture for right-sided catheterizations
c. Cinography of the flow of dye through the coronary arteries
d. Pressure readings of the various chambers

6. Regina, age 16, is going for a cardiac catheterization, right-sided and left-sided, this morning. She is on digitalis and a no-added-salt (NAS) diet. Which of the following is *not* a usual nursing action in preparing Regina for the cardiac catheterization?

a. Checking to see if all ordered laboratory reports are on the chart, such as PT, PTT, and Hct
b. Keeping her on n.p.o. status and withholding all oral medicines
c. Explaining that she will be awake and that she will be asked to do such maneuvers as coughing and deep breathing during the procedure
d. Allowing Regina to wear her glasses and a watch to the cardiac catheterization laboratory

7. Regina was given 50 mg of hydroxine (Vistaril) and 0.4 mg (gr. 1/150) of atropine sulfate intramuscularly (IM) before the cardiac catheterization procedure. The desired effect of atropine in relation to cardiac catheterization is to

a. Promote sedation
b. Decrease respiratory secretions
c. Prevent bradycardia
d. Eliminate gastrointestinal spasms

8. Regina, age 16, has just returned from the cardiac catheterization lab. She had a right-sided and left-sided (left femoral artery was used) catheterization with no complications, except a minor arrhythmia during the procedure. Her vital signs are stable. Which nursing action is unnecessary for the first hour that Regina is back on the unit?

a. Turning her on her side to give her a backrub
b. Offering her something to drink and telling her fluids help eliminate the dye
c. Checking the pulses distal to the left femoral artery and comparing these with the pulses in the right foot
d. Taking her temperature every 15 minutes for three times

REFERENCES

American Heart Association, Committee on Exercise. *Exercise Testing and Training of Individuals with Heart Disease or at High Risk for Its Development: A Handbook for Physicians.* Dallas, TX: American Heart Association National Center, 1975.

American Heart Association Subcommittee on Rehabilitation Target Activity Group. *Standards for Adult Exercise Testing Laboratories.* Dallas, TX: National Center American Heart Association, 1979.

Cogen, R. "Preventing Complications During Cardiac Catheterizations." *American Journal of Nursing* 76: 401–405 (March 1976).

Disch, J. *Diagnostic Procedures for Cardiovascular Diseases.* Norwalk, CT: Appleton-Century-Crofts, 1979.

Edwards, M. & Payton, V. "Cardiac Catheterization, Technique and Teaching." *Nursing Clinics of North America* 11: 271–281 (June 1976).

Finesilver, C. "Reducing Stress in Patients Having Cardiac Catheterizations." *American Journal of Nursing* 80: 1805–1807 (October 1980).

Janz, N. & Lampman, R. "The Treadmill Stress Test," *Nursing 81* 11: 37–41 (December 1981): 37–41.

Kaiser Permanente Medical Center. "Cardiac Catheterization." *Patient Information Booklet.* San Francisco, CA, 1980.

Kaiser Permanente Medical Center. "Instructions for Exercise Treadmill Electrocardiogram." *Patient Information Sheets.* San Francisco, CA, 1981.

Kinnebrew, M. "Add Paradoxical Pulse to Your Assessment Routine." *RN* 44:32–33 (November 1981).

Luckmann, J. & Sorensen, K. *Medical–Surgical Nursing: A Psychophysiologic Approach,* 2nd ed. Philadelphia: W. B. Saunders, 1980.

Miller, B. & Keane, C. Encyclopedia and Dictionary of Medicine, Nursing and Allied Health. 2nd ed. Philadelphia: W. B. Saunders, 1978.

Phipps, W. et al. *Medical–Surgical Nursing: Concepts and Clinical Practice.* St. Louis: C. V. Mosby, 1979.

Simoons, M. "The Effects of Drugs on the Exercise Electrocardiogram." *Cardiology* 68 (Supplement 2): 124–131 (1981).

Sivarajan, E. & Halpenny, J. "Exercise Testing." *American Journal of Nursing* 79: 2163–2170 (December 1979).

Smeets, J. P. et al. "Prognostic Value of Thallium-201-Stress Myocardial Scintography with Exercise ECG After Myocardial Infarction" *Cardiology* 68 (Supplement 2): 67–70 (1981).

Strong, A. "Caring for Cardiac Catheterization Patients." *Nursing 77* 7: 60–64 (November 1977).

Teasley, D. "Don't Let Cardiac Catheterization Strike Fear in Your Patient's Heart." *Nursing 82* 12: 52–56 (March 1982).

Tucker, S. *Patient Care Standards,* 2nd ed. St. Louis: C. V. Mosby Co., 1980.

Wenger, N. et al. *Cardiology for Nurses.* New York: McGraw-Hill, 1980.

CHAPTER EIGHT

Endoscopic Procedures

Objectives

1. Compare the various procedures possible with fiberscopes and the older nonflexible endoscopes.
2. Describe nursing assessments for six possible complications, which may occur after endoscopic procedures.
3. Compare and contrast the nursing interventions before and after patients have bronchoscopies, gastroscopies, or other endoscopic procedures involving the upper airway.
4. Identify areas for patient teaching about sigmoidoscopy and other endoscopic procedures of the lower gastrointestinal tract.
5. Identify endoscopic procedures requiring standard pre- and postoperative care due to general anesthesia.
6. Describe nursing interventions for a patient after a cystoscopy, under local anesthesia.

Endoscopes are used for direct visualization of hollow organs or body cavities. Specifically designed endoscopes are named for the cavity that is being viewed, such as a gastroscope, bronchoscope, or sigmoidoscope. See Table 10 for a complete list of endoscopic procedures. The scopes contain lights so that the interior or cavity of the organ can be seen. The scopes are hollow instruments with suction tips, biopsy forceps, and other accessories for obtaining tissue samples. Electrodes for cauterization may also be an accessory. Cameras are used to record the findings for later reference.

Earlier scopes were all rigid instruments, but newer models are flexible nylon tubes, which can more easily be advanced into a body cavity, say, the intestinal tract. Fiberscopes or fiber-optic scopes are made of strands of glass fibers, which reflect light and actually make it possible to see around corners. A flexible fiberscope can be threaded from the mouth into the duodenum (duodenscopy) or from the rectum through the ileocecal

TABLE 10. AREAS VISUALIZED BY ENDOSCOPIC PROCEDURES

Name of Procedure	Area Visualized[a]
1. Arthroscopy	Knee joint
2. Bronchoscopy	Bronchial tree
3. Colposcopy	Vagina and cervix (see Chapter 6)
4. Culdoscopy	Female pelvic organs
5. Cystoscopy	Urinary bladder
6. Endoscopic Retrograde Choledocho-pancreatography (ERCP or ECPG)	Common bile duct and pancreatic duct
7. Enterostomy	Upper colon and small intestine
8. Esophagoscopy	Esophagus
9. Esophagogastroduodenoscopy (EGD)	Esophagus to small intestine
10. Fetoscopy	In amniotic sac to view fetus (see Chapter 9)
11. Gastroscopy	Stomach
12. Laparoscopy	Abdominal cavity
13. Proctoscopy	Anus and rectum
14. Sigmoidoscopy	Sigmoid colon

[a]*Preparation discussed in this chapter unless noted.*

valve into the small bowel (enteroscopy). The first fiberscopes were used in the early 1960s. (Industry also uses fiber-optic instruments to peer into cavities such as automobile engines so that the engine does not have to be dismantled (Hirschowitz, 1979)).

POSSIBLE COMPLICATIONS FROM ENDOSCOPIC PROCEDURES

Although endoscopic procedures cause some pain and discomfort, topical anesthetics make the procedure tolerable for an alert, cooperative patient. An endoscopic procedure may save the patient the risk and expense of a surgical procedure, under general anesthesia. Specific complications for the different types of endoscopic procedures will be covered later, but there are at least five possible risks from any type of endoscopic procedure. These five major risks are:

1. The possibility of perforation of the organ or cavity being scoped.
2. Aspiration of saliva or gastric contents when the upper airway or esophagus is being scoped.
3. Untoward reactions to the drugs used, which include topical anesthetics and medications such as meperidine (Demerol) and diazepam (Valium). Narcotics, tranquilizers or other sedatives may be used both before the test and during the test to help relax the patient. The major side effects of the above drugs are respiratory depression and hypotension. Other specific drugs may also be used during the scope and can cause other side effects.
4. Cardiovascular problems, such as arrythmias and even myocardial infarction, can occur due to the psychological and physical stress of the procedure. A vaso-

vagal effect can be stimulated. The vagus can cause bradycardia because the effect of the vagus is to slow the heart.

5. Hemorrhage can occur, particularly if a biopsy has been done as part of the diagnostic scope.

Transient bacteremia may also occur. The danger of this bacteremia is further explored in the section on cystoscopes. The risks of these complications are low and the exact rates of occurrence depend on the skill of the clinician doing the procedure, the physical status of the patient and the type of instrumentation used (Salmon, 1974).

GENERAL PRETEST NURSING IMPLICATIONS

Data on Chart

Because of the possible risks mentioned above, the physician has the patient sign a special consent form. This form should be on the patient's chart before any sedative medications are given. Baseline studies, hematocrit and urinalysis are routine in most clinic and inpatient settings. Coagulation studies (i.e., partial thromboplastin time (PTT) and platelet studies) are needed if bleeding is a potential problem. If the patient has had any other diagnostic tests before the endoscopy, those results should be available on the chart.

Relieving Pretest Anxiety

Because the patient will be awake during the procedure, he or she should understand the general procedure. As emphasized in Chapter 6, most patients particularly want to know how the procedure ''feels'' (Johnson & Rice, 1974). Some patients may want a detailed explanation of the technical aspects, others do not. Patients should also be told what causes the sensations—if they know what to expect they are less likely to misinterpret the experience. Physical sensations should be described but not evaluated by the nurse because this may create more anxiety (McHugh et al., 1982).

Because the endoscopy is done in a specialized procedure room or operating room, the nurse is usually not present during the actual procedure. Thus, the nurse performs his or her anxiety relieving function well before the patient goes for the exam. As with other diagnostic tests, the nurse can reinforce the information given by the physician and try to find out answers to those questions that continue to bother the patient about the test. Nurses who work in the procedure rooms will have specific functions during the test. Beck (1981) describes the specific roles of the nurse in the endoscopic laboratory.

Physical Preparation of the Patient

With the exception of sigmoidoscopy and culdoscopy (vagina visualization), all the endoscopic procedures discussed in this chapter require that the patient maintain n.p.o. status. Vital signs must be taken as baseline data, and a notation should be made of the patient's general physical status before the exam, e.g., a patient may have abdominal cramps before the exam or shortness of breath. Any preprocedural complaints should be documented in the nurse's notes. The patient should be informed of the frequency of routine vital signs after the procedure so that he or she will not be alarmed by the frequency of the assessments done after the procedure. The patient should void before the procedures so he or she will not have to urinate during the procedure. The patient should be told that the premedications used may make him drowsy and/or euphoric or "not himself." If general anesthesia is planned, the patient should be instructed on deep breathing and coughing exercises and other standard postoperative care. The nurse must protect the patient from injury by keeping the patient on bedrest, with side rails up after the premeds are given.

GENERAL POSTTEST NURSING IMPLICATIONS

Assessing for Complications

The frequency of which to record the patient's vital signs is determined by the routine practices discussed for other invasive procedures in Chapter 6. The patient may want to rest, because the procedures are somewhat of an ordeal. The nurse should check for specific complications each time vital signs are taken. The nurse should particularly assess for bleeding if a biopsy was part of the procedure. Unexplained pain can be due to a perforation. The nurse needs to know what medicines were used both pretest and during the test so that untoward reactions can be noted. For example, if diazepam (Valium) and meperidine (Demerol) were given, the effects of respiratory depression and hypotension may become apparent following the test (Salmon, 1974).

Relieving Pain

Mild analgesics may be needed when local anesthetics wear off. Because severe pain could be due to a perforation, any severe or persistent pain should be carefully assessed.

Checking for the Return of the Gag Reflex

For scopes that involve entry via the throat, the gag reflex can be abolished by administration of a topic anesthetic. With flexible scopes, a topic anesthetic may not be needed. The nurse must check to see if a local anesthetic was used. Even though the patient can swallow, he or she may still not have a gag reflex. The return of the gag reflex can be checked by gently touching a tongue blade to the back of the throat. Once the gag reflex returns, the patient is allowed to resume whatever diet is tolerated.

Patient Teaching for Home Care

Any specific instructions for follow-ups, such as sitz baths or warm gargles, should be explained to the patient. If the patient is going home after the diagnostic procedure, he or she needs explicit instructions on symptoms that should be reported immediately to the physician or clinic. The patient should be accompanied by a friend or family member who in addition to driving the patient home, can also be taught what to look for because the drugs used during the procedure can produce some amnesia in the patient.

BRONCHOSCOPY

Description and Purposes: For a bronchoscopy, a lighted bronchoscope is passed into the bronchial tree. A local anesthetic may be sprayed or swabbed on the throat. The patient lies on his or her back with the head hyperextended. The bronchoscope is inserted via the nose or mouth into the trachea and main stem bronchi. The patient must breathe around the tube. This can cause a fear of suffocation. It is very important that the patient be relaxed and not fight the tube. Oxygen may be administered to assist respirations. A visualization of the mucosa of the bronchi shows the surgeon what area needs to be biopsied. Bronchoscopy is also used therapeutically to remove foreign objects or to do deep suctioning. For suctioning, the bronchoscopy may be done at the patient's bedside, but is usually done in the operating room or a specially equipped room. The bronchoscopy is usually done under a topic anesthetic or with some parenteral sedation. Sometimes general anesthesia is used. Bronchograms (Chapter 1) are sometimes done as part of a bronchoscopy when it is necessary to see the outline of the bronchial tree by x-ray.

Pretest Nursing Implications

Completing Routine Preoperative Care. Most institutions have a routine preoperative check list, which is completed before a bronchoscopy. The consent form must be signed. Hematocrit and urinalysis must be done, etc. The patient is kept on n.p.o. status for about six to eight hours before the procedure. The patient may be on expectorants a few days before the bronchoscopy to clear the respiratory tract. Good mouth care is important before the procedure, so that less bacteria are present in the mouth. Dentures must be removed, and the physician must be warned of any loose teeth.

Patient Teaching. During the procedure, breathing is done through the nose with the mouth open. The patient may need time to practice this. The patient will not be able to talk while the bronchoscope is in his or her throat; therefore, the nurse should explain that the patient will have to communicate by hand signals.

Administering Medications. The pretest medications given parenterally usually include atropine (to dry up respiratory secretions), a narcotic, meperidine (Demerol), and a sedative or minor tranquilizer, such as diazepam (Valium). Diazepam is also a muscle relaxant, which helps with the passage of the tube. As noted in the general introduction, respiratory depression can occur.

Posttest Nursing Implications

Assessing and Preventing Respiratory Embarrassment. The patient is kept in a semi-Fowler's position, but may be turned to either side. The patient should not smoke. Tissues and a paper bag are needed for the expectorations. An emesis basin, lined with tissue, may be useful for copious secretions. (Lining the basin makes it much easier to empty.) A suction machine should be available. Some institutions have routine orders for oxygen for four hours postbronchoscopy (Cameron, 1981). Arterial blood gases are used to assess any persistent hypoxemia. Because severe respiratory embarrassment can occur, a tracheostomy set should also be nearby. An absence of breath sounds may indicate a pneumothorax. Subcutaneous emphysema (a collection of air in tissues) can occur if there is a leak in the pleural space. (See the discussion on thoracentesis or pleural taps in Chapter 6.) Some pink-tinged mucus or small amounts of blood in the sputum are not unusual after the bronchoscope, but hemoptysis can signal hemorrhage from a biopsy site.

Interventions to Promote Patient Comfort. The patient should not do much talking. A pad and pencil can be used for communication. Fluids, particularly warm fluids which are soothing, are encouraged once the gag reflex has returned. Keeping the patient well-hydrated (2000 cc in the adult) helps make respiratory secretions less viscous and thus easier to expectorate (Phipps et al. 1979). A gargle with warm saline may help relieve throat discomfort. Throat lozenges may be used, too. A soft diet may be better tolerated if swallowing is painful. The patient may be very anxious to hear the results of the biopsy because this test is often the determinant of whether malignancy of the lung is operable.

Patient-Teaching. If a bronchogram was done (Chapter 1) the patient may be instructed on postural drainage. If dye was used, this is another reason to force as much fluid as is tolerated so the dye can be eliminated quickly.

GASTROSCOPY

Description and Purposes: A gastroscopy may include viewing the esophagus (esophagoscopy), as well as the interior of the stomach. The presence of any ulcers can be verified and a biopsy taken. If the patient has had a gastrointestinal bleed, it may be necessary for the patient to have a gastric lavage to remove the blood so the gastric mucosa can be visualized.

All endoscopic examinations of the upper gastrointestinal tract are performed with the patient in the left lateral recumbent position. The patient can easily swallow the newer flexible instruments and will not gag if relaxed and properly sedated (Grossman, 1980).

There is sometimes retching as the tube is passed, but usually not vomiting. Most physicians give a small dose of diazepam (Valium 5 mgm) and meperidine (Demerol 50 mgm) intravenously just prior to the procedure to help relax the patient. A gastroscopy is done in a specially equipped procedure room or operating room. Note that the older nonflexible gastroscopes required an anesthetic to be sprayed on the throat to prevent gagging and to reduce discomfort (Salmon, 1974). With the newer flexible scopes, even a local anesthetic may not be used. There is, therefore, less danger of aspiration of secretions into the lung. General anesthesia is not routinely used.

Pretest Nursing Implications

The general preoperative preparation is done, including consent forms, lab work, etc. As with a bronchoscopy, it is very important that dentures be removed and the patient checked for any loose teeth. The patient is kept on n.p.o. status for six to eight hours before the procedure. The usual sedatives and narcotics may be given before the procedure, or sedation may be given intravenously in the procedure room. Studies have shown patients require less analgesia and have less tension if they are given sensory information about the procedure (Stiklorius, 1982). Mouthcare is important, but not as critical as with a bronchoscopy because the stomach normally receives bacteria from the mouth area.

Posttest Nursing Implications

The patient may be kept in a semi-Fowler's position or turned to the side to help expectorate any fluids. The standard vital sign routine is followed, as well as careful checking for any signs of gastric bleeding. If a local anesthetic was used, no liquids are allowed until the gag reflex returns (see bronchoscopy care). Warm saline gargles may be used to relieve a sore throat or throat lozenges can be used. The patient may prefer to rest, rather than eat anything even after the gag reflex has returned. Liquids and soft bland food may be needed until the soreness disappears (Tucker et al., 1980). As with other procedures, the use of drugs may cause specific posttest reactions.

ESOPHAGOGASTRODUODENOSCOPY

A special fiberscope may also be passed down into the duodenum. The patient may or may not have his throat sprayed with a local anesthetic. The drugs used for sedation are usually those described in the introduction to this chapter, meperidine (Demerol) and diazepam (Valium). In addition to these two drugs for sedation, atropine may also be given intravenously. Atropine, an anticholinergic drug, controls gastrointestinal spasms because it blocks the vagal effect on the bowel. (Gastrointestinal motility is stimulated by the vagus.) Two side effects of atropine are a dry mouth and possible tachycardia. Atropine can produce tachycardia because it blocks the slowing effect of the vagus on the heart. The nurse needs to be aware of the drugs used before and *during* the procedure so that side effects can be quickly noted. The pre- and postcare of the patient with an esophagogastroduodenoscopy (EGD) is similar to the care for gastroscopy discussed above. The patient may burp large amounts of air after the procedure (Beck, 1981).

ENDOSCOPIC RETROGRADE CHOLEDOCHOPANCREATOGRAPHY

Endoscopic retrograde choledochopancreatography is usually referred to by the initials, ERCP or ECPG. The procedure involves the passage of a flexible fiberscope through the mouth, stomach, and into the duodenum, as for a EGD discussed above. Glucagon is given to decrease peristalsis in the duodenum (Grossman, 1980). When the endoscope reaches the ampulla of Vater, dye is injected to outline the common bile duct and the pancreatic ducts. X-rays are taken of the biliary tree (cholangiogram). The usual precautions before and after an esophagoscopy or gastroscopy are applicable to the scope of the upper gastrointestinal tract. The additional concerns related to the injection of dye into the biliary system are covered in the section on cholangiograms (Chapter 1). Five possible complications from ERCP are acute pancreatitis, cholangitis, pancreatic abscess, drug reactions, and instrument injury (Burdick, 1978). Serum amylase and lipase levels are useful in assessing for pancreatitis.

SIGMOIDOSCOPY OR PROCTOSCOPY

Description and Purposes: Sigmoidoscopes are used to view the lower colon or sigmoid, and proctoscopes are used to view the anus and rectal areas. When the scope is put through the rectal sphincter, the patient has a strong sensation of a need to defecate. The patient is usually in a knee–chest position or lying on the left side with the knees bent

(Sim's position). The knee–chest position is not needed with the newer flexible sigmoidoscope. The flexible sigmoidoscope also causes little discomfort so no sedation is required. Warming the lubricant may make the insertion less uncomfortable. Examination by an experienced endoscopist can take less than five minutes (Grossman, 1980).

Scopes of the lower colon are used to detect and biopsy polyps and tumors. The clinician can sometimes see the exact site of bleeding or the extent of an inflammatory process. Because most of the cancer of the large intestine is in the lower colon, the sigmoidoscopy is a useful detection tool for cancer (Luckmann & Sorensen, 1980). The procedure can be easily done in an office setting.

The American Cancer Society used to recommend a yearly sigmoidoscopy for all people after age 40. The latest recommendation (American Cancer Society, 1980) is an exam every three to five years after age 50, once the person has had two negative sigmoidoscopies a year apart. A digital rectal exam is still recommended as a yearly exam for patients over age 40. Guaiacs of stool are recommended yearly after age 50. (See Chapter 13 in Corbett (1982) for tests for occult blood and cancer detection.) Nurses can help educate the public on the usefulness of rectal exams to detect cancer of the lower colon.

Pretest Nursing Implications

If the patient has been taking iron pills, these are usually discontinued several days before the exam. The patient may have a light meal the evening before the exam and clear liquids the day of the exam. Bowel preparation usually includes two cleansing enemas an hour or two before the exam. A laxative is not given because this may move stool down into the sigmoid area. As a general rule, the patient is not given sedation. The patient may take enemas at home if the sigmoidoscopy is done on an outpatient basis.

Posttest Nursing Implications

The standard routines for vital signs, checking for bleeding, etc. are followed. The patient will probably need to rest for awhile. A warm sitz bath may be relaxing if the condition permits. The patient may have some mild abdominal cramping.

COLONOSCOPY AND ENTEROSCOPY

These procedures use flexible fiberscopes to view the upper colon and small intestine. Sedation is required but not general anesthesia. Glucagon is given intravenously to decrease any intestinal spasms. Food is withheld for six to eight hours and the bowel prep must be extensive. Sometimes polyps are biopsied and cauterized during a colonoscopy. There is a rare risk of a fatal explosion of colonic gases if electrocautery is used in a poorly prepared colon (Grossman, 1980). In a well prepared colon, there is little danger from electrocautery. The patient may be on a clear liquid diet for a day or two before the exam. Laxatives and suppositories will be used as well as cleansing enemas just before the exam. Other nursing implications are similar to those for other endoscopic procedures.

CYSTOSCOPY

Description and Purposes: The cystoscope is passed through the urethra into the bladder so the interior of the bladder can be examined for inflammation, tumors, stones, or structural abnormalities. Small stones may be removed via the cystoscope. Ureteral catheters may be passed into each ureter to obtain samples of urine from the pelvis of each kidney. A radiopaque due may be injected to do a retrograde pyelogram (see Chapter 1). A cystoscope can be done with topic anesthesia, but more extensive procedures require the use of general or spinal anesthesia. The topic anesthetic is in jelly form and is put into the urethra. The discomfort may be similar to a catheterization.

Pretest Nursing Implications

Routine preparations are done in relation to consent forms, vital sign checks, laboratory work, etc. If the patient is to have general anesthesia, he or she should be instructed on routine deep breathing and coughing and other routines for postgeneral anesthesia. The patient is allowed a full liquid diet if the procedure is to be done under a local anesthetic. The patient may be started on prophylactic antibacterials.

Posttest Nursing Implications

Routine Assessments for Bleeding. The standard vital sign routine is followed. Some hematuria is not uncommon, but the patient should be carefully watched for hemorrhage if a biopsy was done. The patient may be on bedrest for up to four hours. If the procedure was done in a urology clinic, the patient and the patient's family should be instructed on these routine assessments and the other pertinent aftercare.

Monitoring Intake and Output. The patient's intake and output (I and O) should be monitored for at least 24 hours. The adult patient should have an intake of 2500 to 3000 ml, unless contraindicated. If the patient does not have a Foley catheter, the nurse must check for the possibility of urinary retention with overflow. Small amounts, 50 to 100 ml frequently, may be a sign of urinary retention with overflow. If the patient has a Foley catheter, it must be kept connected to a sterile drainage system.

Special Care of Ureteral Catheters. The patient may have a ureteral catheter. These catheters are very tiny and are usually fastened on a splint. It is important that there not be any tension on the catheter or any kinking. Nurses do not routinely irrigate ureteral catheters. If the catheter is to be irrigated, only a few cubic centimeters of sterile normal saline are used because the kidney pelvis holds only about 5 cc of urine. Because the kidney pelvis does not have room for much collection of urine, it is very important that the physician be notified if a ureteral catheter is not draining properly.

Detecting Urinary Tract Infections. Patients are sometimes given antibacterials after a cystoscope because of the high possibility of urinary tract infections from the instrumentation. Any break in the tissue of the bladder may let bacteria into the blood stream; consequently, the patient may have chills and fever from a transient bacteremia. This transient bacteremia may be dangerous for the patient with mitral valve disease because bacterial endocarditis can occur (Koepke, 1980). The nurse should have the patient check for any signs of urinary tract infection, such as burning on urination or cloudy, foul-smelling urine. A urinalysis is usually obtained as part of the posttest procedure. See Corbett (1982) for interpretation of routine urinalysis and culture and sensitivity tests.

Reducing Patient Discomfort. The patient may have some pain when urinating (dysuria) and bladder spasms. Sometimes anticholinergic drugs, such as methantheline bromide (Banthine), are given for bladder spasms. Mild analgesics may also be needed. To stimulate voiding, cholinergic drugs, such as bethanecal chloride (Urecholine), may be needed.

LAPAROSCOPY AND CULDOSCOPY

Description and Purposes: An instrument can be used to inspect the pelvic viscera. If the instrument is inserted into the abdomen through a small incision in the lower abdominal wall, the procedure is called a laparoscopy. The procedure is usually done under general anesthesia. Laparoscopic examination is sometimes done to help diagnose infertility (see Chapter 9). Minor surgical procedures and tubal ligations are also done by laparoscopy. Surgery done via the laparoscope is sometimes called "Band-aid" surgery, because the incision, only 1 or 2 cm long, requires a very small dressing.

The culdoscope is an instrument similar to the laparoscope and also permits direct visual examination of the female viscera. The culdoscope is introduced into the pelvic cavity through a very small incision in the vaginal posterior fornix. The woman is placed in a knee–chest position. Culdoscopy may be done under general anesthesia.

Nursing Implications

Because a laparoscopy is usually done under light, general anesthesia the patient needs routine preoperative preparation. A Foley catheter is usually inserted to keep the bladder deflated. Aftercare is the standard care discussed in the beginning of this chapter. If a culdoscopy was done, the woman should not douche or have sexual intercourse until the incision heals, which takes about a week.

COLPOSCOPY

A colposcope contains a magnifying instrument to view the tissues of the vagina and cervix. (Chapter 6 discusses the use of this instrument by nurse practitioners and the nursing care before and after biopsies of the cervix.)

ARTHROSCOPY

Description and Purposes: An arthroscope is a fiberoptic endoscope used to examine the interior of joints. Although other joints can be visualized, the common arthroscopic procedure involves the knee joint. Arthroscopy of the interior of the knee joint can directly reveal injuries to the meniscus as well as other abnormalities. Minor surgical repairs can also be done by use of the arthroscope. General anesthesia is used if surgical repair is anticipated. Arthroscopic surgery is another of the "Band-aid" surgeries, made possible by fiberoptic endoscopes and microscopic surgical instruments.

Nursing Implications

See Chapter 1 for a description on arthrograms, which may be done before direct visualization of the knee joint or in connection with an arthroscopic examination. Pre- and postprocedure care depends on whether the patient has had local or general anesthesia. The complications discussed in the beginning of this chapter are pertinent. In addition, the nurse should assess for any possible infection, which can be serious in a joint. Some patients may be given prophylactic antibiotics when joints are entered to prevent osteomyelitis.

Questions

1. The introduction of the fiberscope was a great boon to endoscopic diagnostic procedures because the fiberscope enabled clinicians to

- **a.** Take a biopsy specimen
- **b.** See around corners
- **c.** Take pictures inside the body
- **d.** Do cauterizing

2. The nurse should assess for all these potential complications from endoscopic procedures *except*

- **a.** Shock due to perforation of a body organ
- **b.** Hemorrhage due to bleeding from a biopsy site
- **c.** Oversedation due to the use of sedatives before or during the procedure
- **d.** Burns from the light on the end of the instrument

3. Mr. Kent is scheduled for a bronchoscopy today. Which of the following preparations is not part of the routine before a patient has a bronchoscopy done under a local anesthetic?

- **a.** Administration of atropine and a sedative
- **b.** Special emphasis on mouth care
- **c.** Explaining to the patient that he should not talk much after the procedure
- **d.** Teaching the patient how to breathe in and out through the mouth with a noseclip on the nose

4. When a patient has had an anesthetic sprayed on the throat, the assessment that determines the patient can have fluids is

- **a.** Ability to swallow without discomfort
- **b.** Presence of gag reflex when a tongue blade touches the back of throat

c. Absence of nausea or abdominal distention
d. Presence of active bowel sounds

5. Patients should be taught that the American Cancer Society's latest recommendation (1980) for routine sigmoidoscopies after two negative exams a year apart is

a. Annually for all people over 40
b. Annually for all people over 50
c. Every 3 to 5 years after age 40
d. Every 3 to 5 years after age 50

6. Standard nursing care following general anesthesia is most often necessary for a patient having a (an):

a. Laparoscopy
b. Enteroscopy
c. Colposcopy
d. Proctoscopy

7. Nursing interventions after a patient has had a cystoscopy under local anesthesia would include all *except;*

a. Putting the patient on I and O for at least 24 hours
b. Checking for urinary retention with overflow
c. Keeping the patient on n.p.o. status for four to six hours after the procedure
d. Assessing for bladder spasms and giving ordered analgesics PRN

REFERENCES

American Cancer Society. *Report on the Cancer-Related Health Checkup*. New York: American Cancer Society, Inc., February 8, 1980.

Beck, M. ''Preparing Your Patient Physically For an Esophagogastroduodenoscopy.'' *Nursing 81* 11: 88–96 (February 1981).

Burdick, G. ''Endoscopic Retrograde Cholangiopancreatography.'' *Arizona Medicine* 35: 655–656 (October 1978).

Cameron, T. ''Fiberoptic Bronchoscopy.'' *American Journal of Nursing* 81: 1462–1464 (September 1981).

Corbett, J. V. *Laboratory Tests in Nursing Practice,* Norwalk, CT: Appleton-Century-Crofts, 1982.

Grossman, M. ''Gastrointestinal Endoscopy.'' *Ciba Clinical Symposia* 32 (3) (1980).

Hirschowitz, B. ''A Personal History of the Fiberscope.'' *Gastroenterology* 76: 864–869 (April 1979).

Johnson, J. E. & Rice, V. H. ''Sensory and Distress Components of Pain: Implications for Study of Clinical Pain.'' *Nursing Research* 23: 203–209 (May/June 1974).

Koepke, J. *Guide to Clinical Laboratory Diagnosis,* 2nd ed. Norwalk, CT: Appleton-Century-Crofts, 1980.

Luckmann, J. & Sorensen, K. *Medical-Surgical Nursing: A Psychophysiologic Approach*. Philadelphia: W. B. Saunders, 1980.

McHugh, N. et al. ''Preparatory Information: What Helps and Why.'' *American Journal of Nursing* 82: 780–782 (May 1982).

Miller, B. & Jeane, C. *Encyclopedia and Dictionary of Medicine, Nursing and Allied Health*, 2nd ed. Philadelphia: W. B. Saunders Co., 1978.

Phipps, W. et al. *Medical-Surgical Nursing: Concepts and Clinical Practice*. St. Louis: C. V. Mosby Co., 1979.

Salmon, P. R. *Fibre-Optic Endoscopy*. London, England: Pitman Medical Publishing Co., 1974.

Stiklorius, C. "Fair Warnings for Patients Facing Esophagoscopy and Gastroscopy." *RN* 45 64–65 (June 1982).

Tucker, S. et al. *Patient Care Standards, 2nd ed*. St. Louis: C. V. Mosby, 1980.

CHAPTER NINE

Diagnostic Procedures Related to Childbearing Years

Objectives

1. Describe basic information a nurse can provide to couples seeking information about infertility tests.
2. Explain patient instruction needed for each of the five basic infertility tests.
3. Describe some basic facts about amniocentesis that are helpful in planning nursing care for a couple, where the woman is to have an amniocentesis for prenatal genetic diagnosis.
4. Name some common genetic diseases that are detected by three types of tests of amniotic fluid.
5. Explain the therapeutic value of amniocentesis in assessment of isoimmune disease (Rh factor).
6. Explain the clinical significance of determining lecithin-sphingomyelin ratio (L/S ratio) and creatinine levels in amniotic fluid.
7. Describe the routine preparation, including patient teaching, for a patient who is to have an amniocentesis done in late pregnancy.
8. Compare and contrast the oxytocin challenge test (OCT) and the nonstress (NST) of antepartal monitoring.

Even the nurse who is not a specialist in maternal child health nursing may at times be called on to assist with diagnostic procedures commonly done during the childbearing years. The intent of this chapter is to give the reader an overview of the diagnostic procedures used to assess the ability to conceive or to carry a fetus to term. The chapter begins with the five basic tests of infertility because the inability to become pregnant is a common problem. The new and rapidly developing technique of amniocentesis for prenatal diagnosis is discussed in regards to tests for chromosome defects, inborn errors of metabolism, and neural tube defects. Two other uses of amniocentesis, evaluation of the severity of hemolysis from the Rh factor and assessment of fetal maturity, are also explained. Some basic information about fetal monitoring is presented at the end of the chapter.

During the childbearing years, many couples suffer disappointments because of the inability to have the longed for "perfect" child. In recent years, nurses have become very involved in helping families deal with unexpected or crisis situation. Leavitt (1982) describes the impact of nurses who do primary prevention for high-risk families. Nurses who contract with the couples for follow-up visits after a family crisis can actually help strengthen the adaptive capacity of a family. The key point is for the nurse to focus on the family as a unit. Whether it is the crisis of infertility, an unhappy report from an amniocentesis test, or the stress of fetal monitoring, the professional nurse can be instrumental in helping the family cope.

The nurse's sensitivity to the needs of the patient undergoing a diagnostic test is important for short-term care as well as for follow-up. For example, when patients are connected to monitors, or undergoing technical procedures, they may begin to feel depersonalized. However, in one study of 50 mothers who had been monitored during labor, none found the monitor depersonalizing. The investigators noted that the nurses did not walk in the room and look at the monitor first—a normal tendency when machines are being used. Rather, the nurse first spoke with the woman and asked her how she was doing. After the personal interaction and after feeling the woman's contractions, the nurse correlated the clinical findings with the readouts from the monitors (McDonough et al., 1981). As more and more diagnostic procedures are used to assess the natural events of child-bearing, the nurse can continue to supply the essential human element of caring.

INFERTILITY TESTING

A growing number of couples in the United States, (estimated as 15% to 20% of all married couples) seek medical help for infertility (Pfeffer, 1980). Birnbaum (1980) gives three possible reasons for an increased focus on infertility tests: 1) the diminished number of children available for adoption because of legalized abortions; 2) a rising incidence of gonorrhea, which can cause pelvic inflammatory disease (PID) and sterility; and 3) the fact that more women are opting to delay pregnancy until they are in their thirties, when reproduction may not be as easy.

Infertility is defined as the inability of a couple to achieve pregnancy after one year of unprotected intercourse. For some couples, such circumstances as past pelvic inflammatory disease, suspected hormone imbalances, or other physical problems indicate sterility may be a problem. If there are no obvious reasons why a couple should not be able to conceive, infertility tests are not advocated until after a year of unprotected intercourse. A nurse can reassure a couple, who seem healthy, that the failure to get pregnant after only a few months is not an indication to too quickly seek medical help.

For some couples, who have tried for much longer than a year to get pregnant, the decision to begin fertility testing may be a difficult one to make. The tests may be costly. They are an invasion into an area that is usually very private. And beginning the tests is, in

TABLE 11. FIVE BASIC TESTS FOR INFERTILITY[a]

Test	Purpose
Basal body temperature recordings	Gives presumptive evidence of ovulation.
Semen analysis	Assessment of number and characteristics of sperm in one ejaculation.
Hormone analysis	Assessment of hormonal imbalances, which may be primary or secondary hypofunction. Some physicians use the endometrial biopsy. (See Chapter 6.)
Postcoital exam (Sims–Huhner)	Assessment of mobility and number of sperm in cervical mucus after intercourse. Also checks characteristics of mucus at time of ovulation.
Hysterosalpingogram	Assessment of tubal patency and any structural defects in uterus or tubes (Rubin's test only tests tubal patency). (See Chapter 1 on hystosalpingogram.)

[a] *See text for explanation of tests and patient teaching.*

a way, an acknowledgment of failure to do something that is thought of as being "natural." Patients may discuss with nurses the frustration in not being able to get pregnant. The nurse can assess if the couple needs a referral for infertility testing. The nurse can stress that infertility may be due to a problem with the male, female, or both; therefore, both people need to be tested, once the couple has decided they need help. A brief explanation of the five basic tests for infertility are summarized in Table 11.

BASAL BODY TEMPERATURE RECORDS

The term basal refers to the lowest possible level of a physiologic measurement (i.e., baseline). The basal body temperature (BBT) is taken early in the morning before the woman gets out of bed. Because this test requires only a thermometer and a graphic chart, women may do this test before they seek medical advice. If the woman can determine her ovulatory pattern, the couple can plan intercourse to take advantage of her fertile period. (Using a temperature chart to avoid conception is not always reliable because the change in temperature is associated with ovulation, not before.)

In females who have a normal menstrual cycle, the basal temperature is usually below 98°F (36.7°C) in the preovulatory phase. Before ovulation occurs, an increasing production of estrogen may cause a slight downward trend in the basal temperature. Then with ovulation, the "other female hormone," progesterone, is secreted by the corpus luteum. Progesterone affects the hypothalmus so there is up to a degree rise in the basal temperature. The increase in temperature at ovulation usually makes the woman's basal temperature above 98°F (36.7°C). If the woman accurately keeps a graphic recording for a few months, a physician can interpret the charts and note if there is presumptive evidence that ovulation is occurring. The patient needs to note on the chart any colds or infections, which would disrupt the normal temperature pattern.

Preparation of Patient for Basal Temperature Recordings

The patient should be instructed on exactly when to take the temperatures and how to record them on the graph. (Nurses seem to forget that shaking down a thermometer, reading the results in tenths, and plotting the number on a graph are skills that may need to be learned.) The woman should be given the chance to practice any of the necessary skills of which she is unsure. Each morning as soon as the patient wakes up, she should take and record her temperature. The woman should be instructed to take the temperature before she goes to the bathroom or does any physical activity, including sex. Oral temperatures are usually sufficient. The patient is given a special chart to record the temperatures, which is brought back to the physician's office or infertility clinic to be analyzed.

SEMEN ANALYSIS

An investigation of semen is the most important initial diagnostic study of the male. If the analysis seems normal, more intensive investigation of the female is in order. In the laboratory a sperm count is done as well as an examination of the form of the sperm, its mobility, and the amount and characteristics of the semen. If any abnormalities are noted or if the count is low, a second specimen will be examined because there are variations with each ejaculation.

Preparation of Patient and Collection of Sample

The patient needs specific instructions on how to collect the specimen. Semen is collected after two or more days of sexual abstinence. The patient may be given privacy in a bathroom to collect the specimen in a jar by masturbation. Obviously, this is a highly intimate matter and creates tension and anxiety in the man. Some men, for psychological or religious reasons, prefer to collect semen at home by using a condom during intercourse. The condom should not contain lubricants or substances that may interfere with the analysis. The patient may be given a plastic sheath to use as the condom. (Religious practices may necessitate a small puncture in the sheath.) All of the semen is put into a clean jar. It must be sent to the laboratory within two hours after ejaculation.

Reference Values:

- 20 to 40 million sperm per ml
- Semen volume of 2 to 5 ml
- Sperm motility 60 percent (within two hours of collection)

POSTCOITAL EXAMINATION: SIMS–HUHNER TEST, HUHNER TEST

The Sims–Huhner test is an examination of the number and motility of the sperm found in the cervical mucus of the woman after intercourse. The test is done a day or two before expected ovulation because an increased secretion of estrogen causes certain characteristic changes in the mucus. Normally, these mucus changes enhance sperm survival. (Learning the mucus changes for ovulation is the basis for a form of contraception called the Billings method.) The postcoital examination can help determine if there is any immunologic or hormonal problems contributing to the infertility.

Preparation of Patient and Collection of Sample

The test is planned for a day or two before the woman's expected time of ovulation. The couple has intercourse, and the woman then goes to the clinic or office for a pelvic examination. The woman may be told to stay in bed for about half an hour after intercourse. The sample of cervical mucus needs to be obtained two to four hours after intercourse. The couple should not use any lubricants, and the woman should not douche. (These instructions may seem obvious, but the health professional must make sure that the patient really understands the test.)

Reference Values:

The microscopic examination shows the quality of the mucus, including the pattern it makes on a slide. Certain patterns are considered normal. The number and motility of the sperm are observed. Ten or more sperm found per high power field is considered a normal count.

TUBAL PATENCY TESTS, HYSTEROSALPINGOGRAM AND TUBAL INSUFFLATION (RUBIN'S TEST)

The tubes can be insufflated with carbon dioxide (Rubin's test) or radiopaque dye (Hysterosalpingogram) to see if the tubes are patent. Instillation of carbon dioxide can be done in the physician's office, but it does not give the detailed information that the dye does. Hysterosalpingogram is very useful for observing any structural defects in the uterus or tubes. A hysterosalpingogram is done in the radiology department. (See Chapter 1 for the discussion on nursing implications of a hysterosalpingogram.)

Hysterosalpingogram or the Rubin's test may also have a therapeutic effect because they break up adhesions in a tube or remove debris that was blocking the tube (Shane et al., 1976).

MEASUREMENT OF HORMONES

The levels of FSH and LH, as well as testosterone, progesterone, and estrogen, may be assessed by laboratory tests to determine normal hormonal balance in both the male and the female. Some physicians prefer an endometrial biopsy to determine the quantity of progesterone rather than serum levels of the hormone (Pfeffer, 1980). An endometrial biopsy can be done as part of a cervical exam (see Chapter 6).

NURSE'S ROLE IN HELPING WITH TREATMENTS

Laboratory tests may or may not be sufficient to identify the cause of infertility. Depending on the results of the basic tests, the physician may order other tests, such as laparotomy to examine the female reproductive organs in more detail (see Chapter 8). Surgical reconstruction may be needed. For women who are not ovulating, medications such as clomiphene (Clomid) may be prescribed by the physician. The nurse's role will depend on the particular treatments tried. Friedman (1981) describes the role of the nurse in a private infertility practice and the many available options for therapy. Obstetric textbooks, such as Olds et al. (1980) or Jensen et al. (1981) also discuss standard treatments, some of the ethical and legal issues, and the role of the nurse in treatments for infertility.

FINDING ALTERNATIVES TO BIOLOGIC CHILDBEARING

Although treatment can help many infertile patients, the success rate for all infertility patients, irrespective of etiology, is approximately 50 percent in most centers (Shane et al., 1976). These statistics mean little or nothing to the individual couple, but they do have implications for counseling because for many couples infertility cannot be presently treated. The final pronouncement of it being highly unlikely that a couple can have a biologic child is a difficult fact for many couples to accept. Adoption may or may not be the answer for a couple. Unusual solutions such as "surrogate mothers" are being tried by some couples when the male is fertile. Couples may benefit from talking to other couples who have been unable to conceive. There are various support groups for infertile couples. The nurse can find out if there is a support group in a local area. The individual who has an infertility problem may feel guilt over the perceived "inadequacy." If the couple does not remain a couple, the individual may have problems explaining this infertility to a new partner.

ALLOWING THE EXPRESSION OF GRIEF AND MOURNING

The loss of a child, either real or desired, does cause a period of grieving. Wong (1980) has written about the empty-mother syndrome. Although Wong's work has been with mothers who have lost children after a lengthy illness, the four interventions she has used to help resolve grief may be applied to several situations discussed in this chapter, including infertility, the birth of a defective child, or the termination of a pregnancy. Interventions to help relieve grief can include 1) preparing the couple for anticipating *normal* feelings of emptiness, loneliness, and failure; 2) helping the couple reevaluate their roles in a childless family (or in a family that does not have the perfect or longed-for child); 3) encouraging the couple to explore fulfilling activities, which utilize their special talents and abilities; and 4) supporting the couple by helping them to communicate with each other and with other family members who have been affected by the loss of a child (Wong, 1980, p. 389), for example, potential grandparents can be very hurt by the lack of a grandchild so they too need help to express their feelings of loss. Obviously the meaning of the loss is very individualized and varies tremendously from situation to situation.

SCREENING TESTS DONE DURING PREGNANCY

The introduction of "the Pill" gave women more control deciding when or whether to have a child. Also, as women's roles have changed in America, more women are opting to have children at a later age—after a career is established. The media is full of stories about women who postpone babies until their thirties. For example, in *McCall's* magazine, the question "How old is too old to have a baby?" is answered with a quote from a physician who says, "When you quit menstruating" (Pines, 1980). The use of amniocentesis and other advanced techniques have increased the probability of healthy normal babies for what used to be called elderly (over age 35) primigravidas. Amniocentesis and various screening techniques have also made it possible for couples, who may be at high risk for genetic defects, to undergo a pregnancy knowing that certain defects can be detected by laboratory testing. Nurses need to be aware of some of the basic things amniocentesis and genetic counseling can offer prospective parents because people often ask nurses for referrals and information on newer trends in health care. The American College of Obstetricians and Gynecologists (1977) recommends genetic counseling for 1) women over age 35, 2) couples who already have one child with a genetic defect, 3) couples with a family history of genetic defects, and 4) couples from ethnic or racial groups at high risk for genetic disease. Corbett (1982) discusses the genetic diseases that are currently being screened by laboratory tests. Note that the Department of Health and Human Services has up-to-date information on genetic tests via the National Clearinghouse for Genetic Diseases.

AMNIOCENTESIS

Purposes: Amniocentesis is the removal of some amniotic fluid for diagnostic purposes. (Amniocentesis can also be done to introduce urea or another hypertonic solution into the amniotic fluid in order to cause an abortion.) The three major reasons for doing amniocentesis for diagnostic purposes include 1) prenatal detection of genetic disorders, 2) follow up and possible treatment of isoimmune disease with the Rh factor, and 3) assessment of fetal maturity. See Table 12 for a summary about the different purposes of amniocentesis.

AMNIOCENTESIS FOR PRENATAL DIAGNOSIS OF GENETIC DEFECTS: THREE MAJOR ASSESSMENTS

Karyotyping for Chromosome Study

A variety of diseases can be detected through a study of the cells and chemicals in the amniotic fluid. Identification of the chromosomes is called karyotyping. A karyotyping of chromosomes is a pattern of the 22 pairs of autosomal chromosomes and one pair of sex

TABLE 12. THREE MAJOR PURPOSES OF AMNIOCENTESIS

Purposes	Timing	Results	Usual Follow-Up
1. Assessment of genetic defects	15th to 18th week of gestation		
a. Karyotyping of chromosomes		Can identify Down's syndrome and other chromosomal abnormalities	Takes 3 to 6 weeks to get all results Couple may opt for abortion if serious genetic defect found
b. Biochemical defects		Over 60 defects can be identified	
c. Alpha-fetoprotein levels		May indicate improper closure of neural tube	
2. Assessment of isoimmune disease (RH factor)	After 24–25 weeks gestation	Level of bilirubin in amniotic fluid indicates severity of hemolysis	Increasing levels of bilirubin may indicate need for intrauterine transfusions or induced labor
3. Assessment of fetal maturity	Near end of gestation		
a. Lecithin/sphingomyelin ratio		Ratio of 2:1 is usually evidence of lung maturity	Labor may be induced if tests indicate mature fetus
b. Creatinine levels		Level of 2 mg/dl is evidence of maturity of kidneys	
c. Staining of fat cells		Evaluate fetal maturity by fat cells	

chromosomes: XX of the female or the XY of the male. All the severe chromosomal abnormalities can be detected by fetal karyotypes. Trisomy of chromosome 21 (Down's syndrome) is the most common abnormality found. The American College of Obstetricians and Gynecologists (1977) states that the risk of Down's syndrome is 1:100 in women over age 40. Although other sources may give various statistical rates for Down's syndrome, most centers routinely offer genetic counseling services to any woman over the age of 35 because there is general agreement that the incidence of Down's syndrome increases with increasing maternal age. Amniocentesis is also offered to women who have had one child with a defect or have a family history of chromosomal defects.

If there is a possibility of a sex-linked defect such as hemophilia, the sex of the baby may be important. Some diseases, such as hemophilia, are linked to the X chromosome; therefore, if the fetus is a female, there is little if any possibility of the disease. The hemophilia trait is transmitted by the female and occurs in males. A female must have two defective X chromosomes, which is a very rare possibility. Although the sex of the baby is always determined with the chromosomal study, the parents may prefer to not know the results unless there is a possibility of a sex-linked disease. Centers inform the prospective parents that they can know the sex if they so desire.

Biochemical Defects

At least 60 enzyme or biochemical abnormalities can be detected by amniocentesis (Hogan & Tcheng, 1978). Some of the metabolic diseases tested for are galactosemia, maple syrup urine disease, Gaucher's disease, and Tay–Sachs disease. Some of these diseases will only be tested if it is known that both parents are carriers. For example, Tay–Sachs can be detected in the carrier state in parents and because the disease is caused by a recessive gene, both parents must be carriers in order for the fetus to be at risk. Some of the common genetic metabolic defects, such as cystic fibrosis, PKU, and sickle cell anemia, cannot currently be tested by study of the cells in amniotic fluid. See Corbett (1982) for laboratory tests of carrier states for biochemical defects.

Alpha-Fetoprotein Levels to Detect Neural Tube Defects

Alpha-fetoprotein (AFP) is manufactured by the fetal liver. Normally, there is a low level of this protein in the amniotic fluid, but if the neural tube does not close properly, large amounts of AFP leak into the amniotic fluid (Kimball et al., 1977). If the neural tube does not enclose at the top, the fetus fails to develop a normal brain (anecephaly). If the defect in the neural tube is lower, the fetus has spinia bifida. A meningocele or myelomeningocele may be associated with the spinal bifida. The more involvement of the spinal cord, the more severe the handicap. The child may be paralyzed from the waist down, have the lack of bowel and bladder control, or the damage may be slight and amenable to therapy. Severe omphalocele (inversion of internal organs) or congenital nephrosis can also cause increased levels of AFP. If the amniotic fluid is contaminated with fetal or maternal blood, the AFP level may be falsely high because the protein is normally high in the blood. Twins will also cause increased levels of AFP in amniotic fluid. As with other tests of amniotic fluid, the physician must make interpretations cautiously based on as much data as possible. Some of these structural defects may also be identified by ultrasound tests (see Chapter 4).

ALPHA-FETOPROTEIN IN THE SERUM

By about 16 to 18 weeks of pregnancy, alpha-fetoprotein can be measured in the mother's blood. Note that currently a maternal blood test for AFP is the *only* screening test that can be done of the pregnant woman's blood as a check for genetic defects in the child. (Several defects can be tested by fetal blood samples, as will be discussed later.)

Unfortunately, high levels of AFP in pregnant women do not always indicate a problem with neural tube defects because there may be an incorrect estimation of the fetal age, twins, or other reasons for an increase, which are not well understood yet. Still, even with these drawbacks, AFP blood screening is being offered to pregnant women in certain screening programs in the United States. Alpha-fetoprotein screening is already being routinely done in other countries, such as England and Australia. If the AFP blood screening test is elevated, a repeat is done. If the test is positive on a second blood sample, the woman has an ultrasonogram (Chapter 4). If there is still doubt about the possibility of a defect, an amniocentesis is done.

Because AFP blood testing is the first large scale screening test offered to any woman, there are concerns about how the test will be conducted and if the couple will have the benefit of informed advice. At the present time, the proposed FDA regulations are that the sale of AFP materials to laboratories should be available only when physicians are participating in comprehensive screening programs (Chedd, 1981). It will be interesting to see what develops with AFP as the first maternal blood test to screen for genetic disease. Opponents of mass screening say that testing of all pregnant women causes a great deal of unnecessary anxiety, particularly if one is opposed to terminating the pregnancy.

Counseling before an Amniocentesis for Prenatal Diagnosis

Although the technical preparation of the patient for amniocentesis is very simple, the psychological care of the patient may be very complex. Tishler (1981) described in detail the psychological aspects of genetic counseling. If amniocentesis is being done for genetic counseling, the bottom line is "what action will be taken if there is an abnormality found?" Counseling is done before the amniocentesis to help the couple fully understand the ramifications of the test so they can make an informed decision. If the couple has no desire to terminate the pregnancy, most centers advise against having an amniocentesis because it does not change the course of events. (At the present time, treatment or correction is not usually feasible in utero. The exception is for isoimmune problems, which will be discussed later.)

Although amniocentesis is considered to have very little risk for the mother and less than 1 percent risk for the fetus, the couple must be aware of the possibility of damage or death to the fetus. The physician in a particular center or a genetic counselor, who may be a nurse or other health professional, can explain the statistics of a particular center.

Although a couple may not want to agree to terminate a pregnancy if the results show a defect, they may desire the amniocentesis to better plan for the birth of a defective child. The nurse who works in a setting where amniocentesis is done must be aware of the hard decisions couples must make about whether the findings from an amniocentesis are reason for an abortion. Pressures from family and friends, and society in general, may make it difficult for the couple to choose what is right for them.

A genetic counselor can be invaluable in supplying the couple with correct data to help them make their own decision. Obviously, there are several bio-ethical issues that are raised when prenatal diagnosing is done. Chedd (1981) discusses not only the broad ethical issues of genetic screening but also the legal problems that can arise. Surely this is an area that will spark even more legal and ethical arguments in the future as more women take advantage of amniocentesis.

Timing of Amniocentesis and Waiting for the Results

An amniocentesis for prenatal diagnosis is usually done between 14 and 18 weeks of gestation. Before this time, there is not enough fluid and cells for a culture. The results of the test take three to six weeks because of the need to culture cells to do chromosome patterns (karyotyping) and metabolic studies. This waiting period is a time of extreme anxiety for most couples. The woman may be trying to conceal the pregnancy until she knows the fetus is all right. (A pregnancy of 20 or more weeks is difficult to conceal.) The couple tend to have very ambivalent feelings about the fetus because it is possible that it may be aborted. Crying and indecision about the pregnancy are common feelings. If the results indicate a serious defect and an abortion is done, the abortion must be by induction because the patient is in the second trimester. Happily, the most common result of an amniocentesis is a *prediction* of normality. It is important that couples understand not all possible defects are tested by amniocentesis and there is always a possibility of error. The fact is stressed that no test can *guarantee* a healthy baby. But for a couple with reason to fear one of the defects that can be identified by amniocentesis, a report of no defect is joyous news. The woman who does not have the support of the father of the child may have an even more difficult time awaiting the report of the amniocentesis.

AMNIOCENTESIS IN ISOIMMUNE DISEASE (Rh FACTOR)

Amniocentesis for follow-up of isoimmune disease is not done before 24 to 25 weeks gestation because intrauterine transfusions are impractical before this time (Olds et al., 1980). If the mother has a rising titer of Rh antibodies, the amniocentesis may be done several times during the pregnancy to monitor the welfare of the fetus. (A rising bilirubin level in the amniotic fluid indicates hemolysis of fetal red blood cells.) Elevated or rising Rh antibody titers in the mother indicate that the fetus may have hemolytic disease of the newborn (HDN). This disease, formerly called erthyroblastosis fetalis, was even more common before the introduction of immunoglobulins of Rh antibodies (RhoGam), which can be given in certain cases to prevent the mother from making antibodies against the Rh factor of the fetal cells. (RhoGam is used within 72 hours after each pregnancy of a Rh negative mother with a Rh positive infant.) Other isoimmune factors, such as ABO incompatibility, can cause some hemolytic reactions, but it is the Rh factor that causes the severe increase in bilirubin due to massive hemolysis of the red blood cells of the fetus. In some institutions if an indirect Coomb's test, which measures antibody titers in the pregnant woman's serum, goes above 1:16, amniocentesis is done to determine the severity of the hemolytic disease in the fetus (Jones, 1975).

Reference Values

The amount of bilirubin in the amniotic fluid is measured by how it changes patterns of light at a certain wave length (spectrophotometry). Charts are available to compare the concentration of bile pigments at different gestational ages.

Clinical Significance

If there is an abnormal amount of bilirubin for the gestational age, the obstetrician must decide whether to do intrauterine transfusions of the fetus or to induce labor. One of the considerations for inducing labor is the maturity of the fetus. (See the L/S test discussed next.) Olds et al. (1980) gives an excellent description of the role of the nurse in helping with exchange transfusions for the fetus and the newborn.

AMNIOCENTESIS FOR ASSESSING FETAL MATURITY

LECITHIN/SPINGOMYELIN RATIO

The Lecithin/Sphingomyelin Ratio (L/S Ratio) is a test for fetal lung maturity. Lecithin and sphingomyelin are two phospholipids found in amniotic fluids, as well as serum. Sphingomyelin, which is associated with nervous tissue, remains at about the same level in the amniotic fluid throughout the pregnancy. Lecithin is a major component of alveolar surfactant. If there is sufficient surfactant to lubricate the alveolar surfaces, the lungs can inflate normally at birth. Without sufficient surfactant, the newborn infant is very prone to develop hyaline membrane disease or respiratory distress syndrome (RDS). Lecithin begins to rise in the amniotic fluid at about 35 weeks gestation. This rise parallels the development of lung maturity. When the lecithin ratio is about double the sphingomyelin level in the amniotic fluid, the lungs are usually mature.

Reference Values

A ratio of 2:1 is strong evidence that the fetus has mature lungs.

Shake Test for L/S Ratio

A quick way to check if there is sufficient lecithin present is to mix equal parts of alcohol and saline with a sample of amniotic fluid and shake the test tube for 15 seconds. If bubbles persist in the sample, it is presumed that adequate lecithin is present. Certain factors may interfere with this test, such as dirty glassware, so the laboratory may also do a quantitative measurement of the lecithin/sphingomyelin ratio.

OTHER TESTS ON AMNIOTIC FLUID FOR FETAL MATURITY

The obstetrician may use various data to assess if it is relatively safe to induce labor. The L/S ratio mentioned above is the most heavily used indicator because if there is evidence of mature lung function the risk of respiratory distress syndrome (RSD) is much decreased. The laboratory can also stain fetal fat cells to assess the maturity of the fetus. Creatinine levels are an indication of maturity of the kidneys. The creatinine level usually begins to rise about 34 weeks of gestation. By 37 weeks gestation the level is 2 mg/dl or above. The interpretation of all the data from amniocentesis requires the skilled judgment of the obstetrician because no one test can be viewed in isolation of the overall clinical picture of the mother and the fetus.

Pretest Nursing Implications

The actual physical preparation of the patient for amniocentesis is the same whether the collection of fluid is for prenatal diagnosis of a genetic defect, to assess isoimmune disease, or to determine if the fetus is mature enough for an induced labor. As noted earlier, detailed counseling is very important if the couple are having the amniocentesis done because of possible genetic defects. Even at the time of the procedure, the couple may need last minute reassurance. If the amniocentesis is being done to determine if transfusions are needed or if labor should be induced, the mother will also need on the spot reassurance of the purpose of the test and how the physician will use the results to make a decision about care. The patient will need to sign a special consent form that indicates that she understands the purposes of the procedure and the potential complications that can occur (see Chapter 6 on consents for invasive tests).

The nurse should take baseline vital signs. If the amniocentesis is being done in late pregnancy, the fetal heart rate should also be monitored for a baseline reading. No premedications are given. Depending on the timing of the procedure, the patient may or may not need a full bladder for visualization by ultrasound. (See Chapter 4 for a detailed explanation of the use of ultrasound in pregnancy.) Ultrasound is used to visualize the placenta. The patient lies in a recumbant position throughout the sonogram process and actual withdrawal of the fluid. The skin of the abdomen is prepped with an iodine solution (Betadine or Iodophor). Because only one needle puncture is used to remove the fluid the physician does not usually use a local anesthetic. (Chapter 6 describes the medications that are used for local anesthesia.) The physician inserts a long needle through the abdominal wall into the amniotic sac and withdraws 20 to 30 ml of amniotic fluid. The patient will feel the stick, but the aspiration is not painful. The fluid sample is placed in clearly marked test tubes. If the specimen is to be tested for bilirubin, the fluid should be collected in a dark tube and protected from the light because light will change the composition of indirect bilirubin. (Light is actually used as a therapy, phototherapy, for high indirect bilirubin in the newborn.) After the needle is withdrawn, a band-aid is put over the puncture site in the abdomen.

Posttest Nursing Implications

If the amniocentesis was done in early pregnancy, for prenatal diagnosis, the patient can go home after the test is completed. The patient may be asked to wait a short time so that vital signs can be assessed. The patient is told she may have some mild cramps for a short time and is given instructions to notify the physician or clinic if severe cramps develop or if bleeding occurs. The genetic counselor will have already impressed on the couple that the results of the test will not be available for several weeks, but the couple should be reminded again that they will be called as soon as the results are known.

If the amniocentesis is done in late pregnancy, to assess the status of the fetus, the patient may or may not be hospitalized. The fetal heart rate is monitored for 30 minutes after the test to assess for any difficulty.

FETOSCOPY

By using a fiberoptic lens, physicians can actually view the fetus while it is still in the uterus. (See Chapter 8 for a discussion on the use of fiberscopes.) This visualization can allow the physician to take samples of blood and skin tissues from the fetus. At the present time, fetoscopy is still in its infancy. When fetoscopy becomes more widely available, this will broaden not only the detection of defects but will also make it routine to do treatments to the fetus. Fetal blood can be tested for Duchenne muscular dystrophy, hemophilia A, and B-Thalassema major (McCormack, 1979). At the present time, attempts to test fetal blood for sickle cell anemia are not always successful because of the amount of fetal hemoglobin present. The reader is encouraged to consult recent literature for the latest advances in fetoscopy.

FETAL MONITORING NONSTRESS TEST

Fetal monitoring, a noninvasive technique to evaluate the status of the fetus, is called the nonstress test (NST) to distinguish it from the oxytocin challenge test (OCT), which does put stress on the fetus. The mother is attached to a fetal monitor and the fetal heart rate (FHR) is recorded. The specific patterns of fetal heart rate acceleration and deceleration are classified as abnormal or normal responses to stimuli.

Pretest Nursing Implications

The test may be done in a clinic, office, or in a quiet room in an obstetric unit. The patient is put in a recliner chair or a comfortable bed. The patient should void before the procedure so she will remain comfortable. It is also advisable for the patient to eat before the test because the active bowel sounds of an empty stomach may interfere with the test. The nurse should take a baseline blood pressure. The monitors are applied per hospital routine. The sleep–awake pattern of the fetus is observed for about 40 minutes because a rest–activity pattern of the fetus is usually in a 20 to 40 minute pattern (Lieber, 1980). Some women may have to be monitored longer to obtain a reactive pattern. If the mother is on any sedative drugs, the fetus may be less active.

Experienced maternal child health nurses may do the entire monitoring procedure. The interpretation of the reading will be done by a physician experienced in antepartal monitoring.

Although the nonstress method of antepartal monitoring does not cause any pain or physical discomfort for the woman, most women are highly anxious about the results. Fetal monitoring is only done on patients where there is a probability of fetal jeopardy such as a mother with diabetes or hypertension or other risk factors (Schuler, 1979). The nurse should allow the woman to ventilate her concerns and anxieties. The nurse can answer any questions the woman may have about her prenatal care or the process of labor and delivery. The nurse can also help the patient use some of the relaxation techniques that she may be learning in childbirth classes. A study of maternal reactions to fetal monitoring revealed that the women wanted the nurse with them much or most of the time. The women in the study wanted "someone to hold onto, someone who cares" (Shields, 1978; p. 211).

OXYTOCIN CHALLENGE TEST

The oxytocin challenge test (OCT) is used to determine the ability of the fetus to withstand contractions prior to labor. Because contractions produce a transient decrease in the utero-placental blood flow, some infants may be stressed by labor. The challenge test may indicate which fetus would be in less jeopardy if a cesarean delivery was initiated. Because there is some risk of inducing labor with this test, the test must be done close to a delivery suite. In a study of 800 OCTs on 300 patients, the complication of induced labor was rare, unless the patient was postmaturity (Diamond, 1978). Oxytocin challenge test is not done if there is threatened premature labor, if there has been a previous cesarean birth, or if the patient has bleeding or abnormalities such as placenta previa (Jensen et al., 1981). The OCT is not done in a pregnancy less than 33 or 34 weeks. Because OCT does have some risks, more qualified personnel are needed to give the test. The OCT takes longer and is more costly than the nonstress method (NST) of antepartal monitoring.

Pretest Nursing Implications

The test is given near a delivery suite. The general preparation of the patient is the same as with the NST except the patient will be asked to sign a special consent form, which explains the possible risks of the procedure. (See Chapter 6 on informed consent.) The usual procedure is to give oxytocin intravenously at a specific dilution ordered by the physician. The drip rate is increased until the mother is having three contractions in 10 minutes. The fetus is monitored for at least 30 minutes. The nurse must carefully monitor the patient during the test. The patient can be helped to go with the contractions by using the techniques she is learning in her childbirth class.

Reference Values

The specific patterns must be carefully evaluated by the physician in conjunction with other clinical data. A negative OCT would show no late deceleration in the fetal heart rate after a contraction. In essence, a negative test is evidence that the fetus is not in jeopardy at the present time and the pregnancy may be allowed to progress normally because the fetus can withstand the stress of labor contractions. Crawley et al. (1978) is an excellent home study continuing education program on fetal and maternal monitoring for the nurse wishing in-depth information.

Questions

1. John and Mary Menendez (both age 27) have been married a little over two years. Although they have used no form of birth control for the past 16 months, pregnancy has not occurred. The couple desire a child so they have asked a nurse in a clinic about infertility testing. Which statement is accurate?

- **a.** Infertility is most likely not a problem because they have only been having unprotected intercourse for a little over a year.
- **b.** Infertility is usually due to female problems so only Mary needs to be tested initially.
- **c.** Most all infertility problems are easily treated with new drugs such as clomiphene (Clomid).
- **d.** Basic infertility tests include semen analysis, postcoital exams, and tubal patency tests such as the hysterosalpingogram.

2. As part of an infertility work-up, Mary is to keep a record of her basal body temperature on a daily basis. The nurse is assessing to see if Mary can accurately read the thermometer. In addition, the nurse should stress

- **a.** The temperature should be taken before Mary gets out of bed in the morning.
- **b.** An increase in temperature is expected before ovulation occurs.
- **c.** Rectal temperatures are the only way to obtain a basal reading.
- **d.** A one month's graph of temperatures will usually suffice.

3. Which of the following statements about amniocentesis is an important fact when planning care for the patient who is to undergo an amniocentesis for prenatal diagnosis of genetic defects?

- **a.** The amniocentesis must be done as early as possible—usually before the eighth week of gestation.
- **b.** The test is a guarantee of a healthy baby.
- **c.** The results take 3 to 6 weeks so this is a period of great anxiety for the couple who may decide to terminate the pregnancy.
- **d.** There is a significant risk of 5 to 10 percent for the fetus.

4. Mrs. Sanders is a 39-year-old primigravida who has elected to have an amniocentesis for prenatal diagnosis. At the present time, which of these following congenital diseases can be definitely identified by chromosomal study (karyotyping)?

- **a.** Cystic fibrosis
- **b.** Sickle cell anemia
- **c.** Hemophilia
- **d.** Down's syndrome

5. One of the tests done on amniotic fluid is a test for fetal alpha protein because an elevation of this protein is evidence of

a. Fetal lung immaturity
b. Immunologic deficiencies
c. Neural tube defects
d. Phenylketonuria

6. Mrs. Ragella is 34 weeks pregnant. An amniocentesis revealed an increased bilirubin level as compared to levels done a week ago. This rising bilirubin level is indicative of

a. Possible fetal jeopardy due to hemolytic disease
b. Normal liver functioning
c. Renal immaturity
d. Fetal distress due to hypoxia

7. The physician is concerned because a too early cesarean delivery may predispose Mrs. Ragella's infant to respiratory distress syndrome (RDS). Which of these tests of amniotic fluid is used to assess lung maturity in the fetus?

a. Lecithin-sphingomyelin ratio
b. Creatinine levels
c. Karyotyping of chromosomes
d. Spectrophotometric analysis of bilirubin levels

8. Mrs. Foster is a diabetic who is near term with her second pregnancy. Her other pregnancy was a still birth. She has been admitted to the obstetric unit for a possible early delivery. She is scheduled for an amniocentesis this afternoon to assess fetal maturity. Mrs. Foster asks the nurse about the procedure. The nurse should explain to Mrs. Foster that

a. Premedication will be used to relax her
b. Local anesthesia must be used to eliminate pain
c. Ultrasound will be done to visualize the placenta and fetus
d. X-ray of the abdomen is routine after the procedure is completed

9. Mrs. Foster is scheduled for more tests. She asks the nurse if an OCT is the same as the routine fetal monitoring she had with her last pregnancy. The nurse should explain that the oxytocin challenge test (OCT) *differs* from the nonstress technique (NST) of antepartal monitoring in that the OCT

a. Requires the fetal heart rate be assessed with internal fetal monitors to detect any abnormal patterns.
b. Uses a drug to cause contractions.
c. Is used for women who have high risk pregnancies.
d. Causes anxiety while the NST is anxiety-free for the mother

REFERENCES

American College of Obstetricians and Gynecologists. *Causes and Treatments for Genetic Disorders*. (Patient Information Booklet) Chicago, 1977.

Birnbaum, S. "Procedures and Prognosis for the Infertile Couple." *Mother's Manual* 16: 14–22 (July/August 1980).

Chedd, G. "The New Age of Genetic Screening." *Science* 81: 32–40 (January/February 1981).

Corbett, J. V. *Laboratory Tests in Nursing Practice*. Norwalk, CT: Appleton-Century-Crofts, 1982.

Crawley, M. et al. "Fetal and Maternal Monitoring" *American Journal of Nursing* 78: 2097–2120 (December 1978).

Department of Health and Human Services. *Human Genetics: Informational and Educational Materials* 1: 1, 1979.

Department of Health and Human Services. *Clinical Genetic Service Centers. A National Listing*, 1980.

Diamond, F. "High Risk Pregnancy Screening Techniques." *JOGN* 7: 15–19 (November/December 1978).

Friedman, B. "Infertility Workup." *American Journal of Nursing* 81:2040–2046 (November 1981).

Hogan, K. and Tcheng, D. "The Role of the Nurse During Amniocentesis." *JOGN* 7: 24–27 (September/October 1978).

Jensen, M. et al. *Maternity Care: The Nurse and the Family*, 2nd ed. St. Louis: C. V. Mosby Co., 1981.

Jones, M. B. "Antepartum Assessment in High Risk Pregnancy." *JOGN* 4: 23–27 (November/December 1975).

Kimball, M. et al. "Prenatal Diagnosis of Neural Tube Defects: A Reevaluation of the Alpha Fetoprotein Assay." *Obstetrics and Gynecology* 49: 532–536 (May 1977).

Leavitt, M. *Families at Risk: Primary Prevention in Nursing Practice*. Boston: Little, Brown and Company, 1982.

Lieber, M. "Nonstress Antepartal Monitoring." *Maternal Child Health Nursing* 5: 335–339 (September/October 1980).

McCormack, M. "Medical Genetics and Family Practice." *American Family Physician* 20: 143–154 (September 1979).

McDonough, M. et al. "Parents' Response to Fetal Monitoring" *MCN* 6: 32–34 (January/February 1981).

Olds, S. et al. *Obstetric Nursing*. Menlo Park, California: Addison-Wesley Publishing Co., 1980.

Pfeffer, W. "An Approach to the Diagnosis and Treatment of the Infertile Female." *Medical Aspects of Human Sexuality* 14:121–122 (April 1980).

Pines, M. "How Old is Too Old to Have a Baby?" *McCalls* 107 (June 1980).

Schuler, K. "When a Pregnant Woman Is Diabetic: Antepartal Care." *American Journal of Nursing* 79: 448–452 (March 1979).

Shane, J. et al. *The Infertile Couple: Evaluation and Treatment. Ciba's Clinical Symposia* 28 (5) (1976).

Shields, D. "Maternal Reactions to Fetal Monitoring" *American Journal of Nursing* 78: 2110–2112 (December 78).

Tischler, C. "The Psychological Aspects of Genetic Counseling." *American Journal of Nursing* 81: 733–734 (April 1981).

Wong, D. "Bereavement: The Empty-Mother Syndrome." *Maternal Child Nursing* 5: 385–389 (November/December 1980).

Answers

Chapter 1

1. b
2. b
3. a
4. a
5. d
6. d
7. b
8. d
9. d
10. a
11. d
12. c
13. d
14. c
15. b
16. a
17. a

Chapter 2

1. c
2. c
3. b
4. a
5. b
6. a
7. d

Chapter 3

1. b
2. b
3. c
4. d
5. b
6. c
7. a
8. a
9. d
10. c

Chapter 4

1. b
2. c
3. c
4. b
5. d
6. d
7. d
8. a
9. b

Chapter 5

1. c
2. d
3. a
4. c
5. d
6. c
7. a
8. d
9. a
10. d
11. d
12. c
13. b

Chapter 6

1. d
2. a
3. d
4. c
5. c
6. a
7. a
8. c
9. a
10. c
11. d
12. b

Chapter 7

1. a
2. a
3. d
4. b
5. b
6. b
7. c
8. d

Chapter 8

1. b
2. d
3. d
4. b
5. d
6. a
7. c

Chapter 9

1. d
2. a
3. c
4. d
5. c
6. a
7. a
8. c
9. b

Appendix

Common Abbreviations Used for Diagnostic Procedure

ABG	Arterial blood gases
AFP	Alpha-fetoprotein
BE	Barium enema
BMR	Basal metabolic rate
CT scan	Computerized axial tomography (*also* CAT)
CSF	Cerebrospinal fluid
ECG	Electrocardiogram (*also* EKG)
ECHO	Echocardiogram
EEG	Electroencephalogram
EGD	Esophogastroduodenoscopy
EKG	Electrocardiogram (*also* ECG)
EMG	Electromyelogram
ERCP	Endoscopic retrograde choledochopancreatography or cholangiopancreatography (*also* ECPG)
FEF	Forced expiratory flow
FEV_1	Forced expiratory volume in one second
FVC	Forced vital capacity
GA	Gastric analysis
GB series	Gallbladder series
GFR	Glomerular filtration rate
GI series	Gastrointestinal series
I-131, I-123, etc.	Radioactive iodine
IVC	Intravenous cholangiogram
IVP	Intravenous pyelogram
KUB	Kidneys, ureters, bladder (flat plate of abdomen)
LP	Lumbar puncture
L/S ratio	Lecithin/spingomyelin ratio
MBC	Maximal breathing capacity (*also* MVV)

MVV	Maximum voluntary ventilation (*also* MBC)
NSR	Normal sinus rhythm
NST	Nonstress test (for fetus)
OCG	Oral cholecystogram
OCT	Oxytocin challenge test
PEG	Pneumoencephalogram
PET	Positron emission tomography
PFT	Pulmonary function tests
RAI	Radioactive iodine
RISA	Radio-iodinated serum albumin (for blood volume)
Tc-99	Technetium (radionuclide)
TV	Tidal volume
UGI	Upper gastrointestinal
VC	Vital capacity
VE	Volume exhaled per minute at rest

Index